Other FAST FACTS Books

Fast Facts for the NEW NURSE PRACTITIONER: *What You Really Need to Know in a Nutshell, 2e* (Aktan)

Fast Facts for the ER NURSE: *Emergency Room Orientation in a Nutshell, 2e* (Buettner)

Fast Facts for the MEDICAL–SURGICAL NURSE: *Clinical Orientation in a Nutshell* (Ciocco)

Fast Facts for the NURSE PRECEPTOR: *Keys to Providing a Successful Preceptorship in a Nutshell* (Ciocco)

Fast Facts for the OPERATING ROOM NURSE: *An Orientation and Care Guide in a Nutshell* (Criscitelli)

Fast Facts for the ANTEPARTUM AND POSTPARTUM NURSE: *A Nursing Orientation and Care Guide in a Nutshell* (Davidson)

Fast Facts for the NEONATAL NURSE: *A Nursing Orientation and Care Guide in a Nutshell* (Davidson)

Fast Facts About PRESSURE ULCER CARE FOR NURSES: *How to Prevent, Detect, and Resolve Them in a Nutshell* (Dziedzic)

Fast Facts for the GERONTOLOGY NURSE: *A Nursing Care Guide in a Nutshell* (Eliopoulos)

Fast Facts for the LONG-TERM CARE NURSE: *What Nursing Home and Assisted Living Nurses Need to Know in a Nutshell* (Eliopoulos)

Fast Facts for the CLINICAL NURSE MANAGER: *Managing a Changing Workplace in a Nutshell, 2e* (Fry)

Fast Facts for EVIDENCE-BASED PRACTICE: *Implementing EBP in a Nutshell, 2e* (Godshall)

Fast Facts About NURSING AND THE LAW: *Law for Nurses in a Nutshell* (Grant, Ballard)

Fast Facts for the L&D NURSE: *Labor & Delivery Orientation in a Nutshell, 2e* (Groll)

Fast Facts for the RADIOLOGY NURSE: *An Orientation and Nursing Care Guide in a Nutshell* (Grossman)

Fast Facts on ADOLESCENT HEALTH FOR NURSING AND HEALTH PROFESSIONALS: *A Care Guide in a Nutshell* (Herrman)

Fast Facts for the FAITH COMMUNITY NURSE: *Implementing FCN/Parish Nursing in a Nutshell* (Hickman)

Fast Facts for the CARDIAC SURGERY NURSE: *Caring for Cardiac Surgery Patients in a Nutshell, 2e* (Hodge)

Fast Facts for the CLINICAL NURSING INSTRUCTOR: *Clinical Teaching in a Nutshell, 2e* (Kan, Stabler-Haas)

Fast Facts for the WOUND CARE NURSE: *Practical Wound Management in a Nutshell* (Kifer)

Fast Facts About EKGs FOR NURSES: *The Rules of Identifying EKGs in a Nutshell* (Landrum)

Fast Facts for the CRITICAL CARE NURSE: *Critical Care Nursing in a Nutshell* (Landrum)

Fast Facts for the TRAVEL NURSE: *Travel Nursing in a Nutshell* (Landrum)

Fast Facts for the SCHOOL NURSE: *School Nursing in a Nutshell, 2e* (Loschiavo)

Fast Facts About CURRICULUM DEVELOPMENT IN NURSING: *How to Develop & Evaluate Educational Programs in a Nutshell* (McCoy, Anema)

Fast Facts for DEMENTIA CARE: *What Nurses Need to Know in a Nutshell* (Miller)

Fast Facts for HEALTH PROMOTION IN NURSING: *Promoting Wellness in a Nutshell* (Miller)

Fast Facts for STROKE CARE NURSING: *An Expert Guide in a Nutshell* (Morrison)

Fast Facts for the MEDICAL OFFICE NURSE: *What You Really Need to Know in a Nutshell* (Richmeier)

Fast Facts for the PEDIATRIC NURSE: *An Orientation Guide in a Nutshell* (Rupert, Young)

Fast Facts About the GYNECOLOGICAL EXAM FOR NURSE PRACTITIONERS: *Conducting the GYN Exam in a Nutshell* (Secor, Fantasia)

Fast Facts for the STUDENT NURSE: *Nursing Student Success in a Nutshell* (Stabler-Haas)

Fast Facts for CAREER SUCCESS IN NURSING: *Making the Most of Mentoring in a Nutshell* (Vance)

Fast Facts for the TRIAGE NURSE: *An Orientation and Care Guide in a Nutshell* (Visser, Montejano, Grossman)

Fast Facts for DEVELOPING A NURSING ACADEMIC PORTFOLIO: *What You Really Need to Know in a Nutshell* (Wittmann-Price)

Fast Facts for the CLASSROOM NURSING INSTRUCTOR: *Classroom Teaching in a Nutshell* (Yoder-Wise, Kowalski)

Forthcoming FAST FACTS Books

Fast Facts for TESTING AND EVALUATION IN NURSING: *Teaching Skills in a Nutshell* (Dusaj)

Fast Facts About the NURSING PROFESSION: *Historical Perspectives in a Nutshell* (Hunt)

Fast Facts for the HOSPICE NURSE: *A Concise Guide to End-of-Life Care* (Wright)

Visit www.springerpub.com to order.

FAST FACTS FOR THE CLINICAL NURSE MANAGER

Barbara J. Fry, MEd (Adult), BN, RN, is president of Workplace Dynamix, Inc., an active member of the College of Registered Nurses in Nova Scotia, and a professional keynote speaker and facilitator. She received a BN and diploma in Teaching in Schools of Nursing from Dalhousie University, Halifax, Nova Scotia, Canada, a Change Management Certificate from Queen's University (1997), and a master of Adult Education from St. Francis Xavier University (2003). Her master's thesis was "Facilitating Workplace Relational Learning: The Intersection of Power, Caring, and Quality of Work Life." As a former staff nurse, nursing instructor, and nurse manager (for 16 years), she inspired a climate of personal excellence and professional competence in the workplace. Drawing on her experience as a nurse manager, healthy workplace relationship consultant, professional speaker, and adult educator, she shares her wealth of knowledge and strategies that work in today's changing health care workplace. She provides leadership in improving quality of work life and facilitates individual and group leadership and accountability for creating healthy workplace relationships. As a powerful, humorous, and inspiring speaker, she was the closing keynote speaker for the Canadian Nurses Association's 100th Birthday Celebration Conference (2008). Today, Ms. Fry continues to advocate and facilitate professionalism in nursing practice and to promote healthy workplace relationships. She is a frequently requested presenter and facilitator in both provincial and national nursing associations.

FAST FACTS FOR THE CLINICAL NURSE MANAGER

Managing a Changing Workplace in a Nutshell

Second Edition

Barbara J. Fry, MEd (Adult), BN, RN

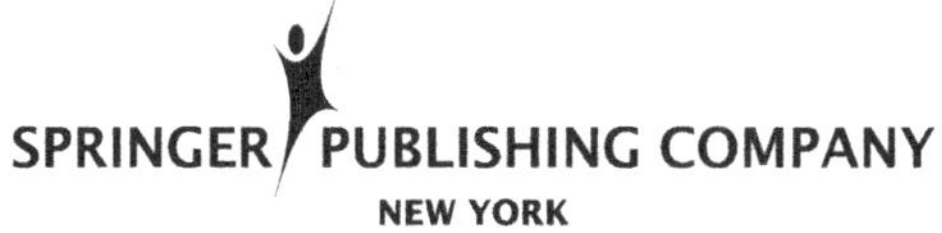

Springer Publishing Company, LLC
11 West 42nd Street
New York, NY 10036
www.springerpub.com

Acquisitions Editor: Joseph Morita
Composition: S4Carlisle Publishing Services

ISBN: 978-0-8261-2788-4
e-book ISBN: 978-0-8261-2789-1

15 16 17 18 / 5 4 3 2 1

The author and the publisher of this Work have made every effort to use sources believed to be reliable to provide information that is accurate and compatible with the standards generally accepted at the time of publication. Because medical science is continually advancing, our knowledge base continues to expand. Therefore, as new information becomes available, changes in procedures become necessary. We recommend that the reader always consult current research and specific institutional policies before performing any clinical procedure. The author and publisher shall not be liable for any special, consequential, or exemplary damages resulting, in whole or in part, from the readers' use of, or reliance on, the information contained in this book. The publisher has no responsibility for the persistence or accuracy of URLs for external or third-party Internet websites referred to in this publication and does not guarantee that any content on such websites is, or will remain, accurate or appropriate.

Library of Congress Cataloging-in-Publication Data

Fry, Barbara, 1948- , author.
Fast facts for the clinical nurse manager : managing a changing workplace in a nutshell / Barbara Fry. — Second edition.
p. ; cm.
Includes bibliographical references and index.
ISBN 978-0-8261-2788-4 (alk. paper) — ISBN 978-0-8261-2789-1 (e-book)
I. Title.
[DNLM: 1. Nursing, Supervisory. 2. Personnel Management. WY 105]
RT89
362.17'3068—dc23

2015033193

Printed in the United States of America by Gasch Printing.

Contents

Part III: Staff Gone Wild? Managing Your Cast of Characters

Part IV: Predicting Your Workplace Future: Create It! Manage It! Love It!

Part V: A Call to Action—From Surviving to Thriving to Recovering the Art of Nursing: Tips and Tools for Managing a Changing Workplace

Preface

Since writing the first edition of *Fast Facts for the Clinical Nurse Manager,* I continued my work delivering keynote addresses, consulting, teaching, and advocating for nurses to work to full scope. I reminded them about the importance of following their standards of practice, to be their professional best, and to be proud of who they are as professionals. As I went about my work, it became obvious to me that many nurses were very worried about their ability to practice to full scope, angry and frustrated about the amount of time spent on completing physical tasks, and concerned about the increasing presence of unregulated staff in practice settings, and that they greatly feared for the future of the nursing profession as a whole. While much was being said in hushed tones and behind closed doors, little was said in the open.

During this time, I experienced three personal "a-ha" moments that reinforced what I was already seeing in practice and hearing from nurses all across Canada. Reflecting on the big picture and energized by my personal experiences, I began to feel a sense of urgency to bring our professional practice issues out into the light of day so they might inspire local, provincial or state, and even national conversations that we have not been having. From these conversations, nurses might begin to see the necessity of taking action to address what we nurses know to be true. I feared that, if we did not begin talking to one another, we could be swept away by care focused exclusively on tasks, leaving other essential aspects of professional nursing care on the back burner. There is enough literature out there to address the negative impact on patient care outcomes and mortality when the full scope of professional nursing practice is absent during the provision of care.

Nursing's issues are longstanding, unresolved, and troubling, and hurt our professional image and patient care. I believe we ourselves are in large part to blame for leaving these issues unaddressed. The interesting thing is that we have the power to change course. Support for nurses is readily available to make the necessary changes now, under the strong leadership of the nurse manager. In order to do so, however, the nurse manager's role must change significantly and quickly. Is there a will to change? Among some managers, I am not sure. Are nurse managers able to change? Yes, given the right professional development opportunities, the desire, and the removal of specific organizational barriers that prevent staff from working to full scope of practice. The latter is perhaps the greatest challenge of all and must spark serious debate. For when organizations fail to create the conditions for nurses to work to full scope, they fail to adhere to the legislation delineating the roles of registered nurse (RN) and licensed practical nurse (LPN). Why are we not having this conversation? Who is lobbying on nurses' behalf? What are nurses saying and doing about this? These are but a few of the questions that arose for me over the past few years and led me, and many more nurses, to the frightening conclusion that, when nurses are not seen to be working to full scope, it is very easy to forget the very powerful and positive role they play in health care delivery worldwide. When they become invisible, they are easily forgotten, and easier and less expensive to replace with unregulated staff or technicians of care. Some would argue that this is okay, but clearly the research says otherwise. Here is a ponderable for you to consider: What would happen in our nations if all the nurses left town (similar to the idea of the television series *The Week the Women Went*)? How well would we fare?

These thoughts coincided with three personally significant events experienced within the past 5 years that launched me on a new professional journey and ultimately led me to write this second edition. They provided the impetus I needed to stop accepting the status quo of sweeping these issues under the carpet and to take the risk of bringing them into the open.

The first event occurred after watching a movie about Florence Nightingale when I suddenly began to weep. The source of my tears both surprised and puzzled me. My thoughts returned to my early days as a new grad, when I held sacred the responsibilities, knowledge, and privilege of being a nurse. My tears, I realized, were of profound sadness about what I believe we have lost as a profession. I was reminded of Hans Christian Andersen's *The Emperor's New Clothes*, in which the observers unite in praise of the emperor's splendid outfit when, in fact, he is wearing nothing at all. Similarly, there is great excitement about all the amazing and wonderful aspects of nursing, yet as many nurses know, despite all the hoopla, there is a darker side that undermines our education, feelings of self-worth, and passion for patient care. What lies beneath must be acknowledged and fixed so that all nurses can thrive in doing the work they are prepared to do for the well-being and health of individuals, communities, and nations.

The second incident registered a deeper, more personal impact when my husband was diagnosed and treated for pancreatic cancer. While he received lifesaving surgery, endured chemotherapy, and underwent numerous readmissions, his physical care by physicians and nurses was beyond reproach. However, he rarely saw the same nurse twice, was asked the same questions repeatedly, and struggled to identify a nurse by name or designation. What shocked me more was that never once was he asked about his concerns or how we were coping as a family. He did not know that this was part of the nurses' role. When I asked him if a nurse sat down to discuss plans for his future care or any other concerns, his comment was, "Oh, they don't have time, they're too busy, but they are really nice." Too busy for a patient with pancreatic cancer, for whom the survival rate is less than 5% after 5 years! His words echoed what I have heard from too many patients and families. I knew then what we have lost as a profession. There was little to no evidence of the nursing process (emphasis on process), continuity of care, or the therapeutic relationship other than "how nice the nurses are." Where was the nursing care plan? In too many of today's practice environments, tasks dominate practice as evidenced by nurses' "To Do" lists or "Cheat Sheets." Nurses do not have enough time to get to know their patients and, for the most part, this is a system issue. (As an aside, after 5 years my husband is considered cured.)

The third event occurred in 2012, when I had an opportunity to visit London, England. While there, I felt compelled to return to my nursing roots and visited the Florence Nightingale museum. Unsure of what I was looking for, an "a-ha" moment soon appeared. Expecting to see the all-too-familiar pictures of the Lady with the Lamp, I quickly became impressed with the extent to which evidence-based practice dominated Nightingale's work. As I continued to absorb the magnitude and impact of nursing's full scope of practice "way back then," the silence of the exhibit was shattered by a hoard of 6-year-old schoolchildren running amok through the museum. They were here to learn about Florence Nightingale by participating in a scavenger hunt and listening to stories about nursing from a real live, elegantly attired "Florence" floating about the museum. I learned that this visit is a requirement of the London school system, serving as a testament to the value placed on professional nursing care. I quickly wondered if there was a lesson here for North Americans and nurses themselves. Like clockwork, the subject comes up about nurses feeling powerless, underappreciated, and devalued, and "wanting to strengthen their voice." Could we do better in advising individual nurses and groups of nurses on how to promote our presence, practice, and professional image? You bet!

Upon my return home, I reflected on my 40-plus years as an RN and the significance of these three previous events. There are numerous pockets of excellence where nurses work to full scope—in particular, community-based programs, family practice, and other specialty areas. In contrast, too many other nurses in other areas of practice struggle daily to overcome organizational barriers, system issues, leadership deficiencies, and feelings of being devalued. It is impossible for nurses to change other people; however, they can have a direct influence on changing systems and how others perceive them. The only person they have the power to change is themselves, and the time has come!

Following these revelations, I knew that nurses need leadership and support to do this and nurse managers have the positional authority and the opportunity to help this happen. Their role requires them to advocate for the conditions necessary for professional practice, and to provide the tools and structures that allow nurses to do the work they were hired to do. Managers have great skills, especially when it comes to managing the relational and professional practice aspects of care provision that take many beyond their comfort zone. Acquiring these additional competencies will help bring managers up to speed and increase their level of comfort in managing today's complex practice environments.

ORGANIZATION

The structure of this book remains similar to the first edition with modifications throughout. Part I addresses the need for nurse managers to change how they manage and lead in a changing practice setting. Chapter 1 introduces evolving leadership and managerial practices. In Chapter 2, nurse managers learn the importance of becoming more political within their organizations. Chapter 3 discusses the new competencies that are no longer on the horizon but present, here and now, for managers and staff.

Part II discusses the reality that change is constant and continues to impact everyone. To that end, nurse managers must be prepared to lead both personally and professionally, sooner rather than later. Thus, Chapter 4 discusses the aura of uncertainty lurking in the corners of every workplace and how to help staff manage it. Chapter 5 addresses the intergenerational staff (the updated, politically correct term!) by deemphasizing generational differences. It touches on diversity, which frequently goes hand in glove with conversations about staff mixes. Chapter 6 takes a lighthearted and broad view of a few popular theories describing the process of organizational change. In Chapter 7, the reader learns what happens when a way of being ends, the impact on staff, and what can be done to help them let go of the past. Then, Chapter 8 describes the chaos and confusion that can erupt when staff members are caught in the middle between the old way and the new. Finally, Chapter 9 points the learning compass to the new way of being.

Part III describes different situations and some of the fascinating characters whom the nurse manager has the privilege of managing. Chapter 10 highlights resistance as a normal part of change and discusses how to manage it. Attitude is the theme of Chapter 11, which reinforces that each of us has the power to choose an attitude that will ultimately affect our personal and collective quality of work life. Chapter 12 addresses one of the toughest challenges nurse managers face—dealing with the toxic impacts of negative behaviors. Finally, Chapter 13 ramps up the previous chapter by tackling the difficult subject of the workplace bully and what to do when there is one on staff.

Part IV discusses the quality of the nurse manager's workplace future and how the manager has the power to create, shape, and significantly influence its direction. The term *work–life balance* is discussed, with an acknowledgment of the influence of recent literature suggesting that creating harmony and a sense of well-being in the workplace and at home is a realistic goal. Chapter 15 identifies the need for developing a mission, vision, and values statement for the practice setting that promotes trust, and creating a team charter as part of a back-to-basics plan. In Chapter 16, the focus is on staff meetings as a vehicle for transformation. Then, Chapter 17 reveals why nurse managers and staff members need a visible presence beyond the confines of their practice setting.

Part V summarizes the main points of the text. Chapter 18 lists the concepts and actions that can give managers a jumpstart and tools for initiating conversations with staff to collaborate in creating a practice setting in which people want to work. Chapter 19 concludes with 10 "Fast Facts" tips for thriving in a changing workplace and 12 more for managing it.

CONVERSATION GUIDES AND ACTIVITIES

The conversation guides and tools included in the Appendix can be modified to fit the needs of staff and are meant to facilitate discussion using small-group and large-group formats.

SUMMARY

This second edition of *Fast Facts for the Clinical Nurse Manager: Managing a Changing Workplace in a Nutshell* is a continuation of observations made through my consultative practice and responses to topics requested for keynote addresses. Although more is being done by some organizations to support the role of the nurse manager, many managers continue to feel adrift and struggle to keep their heads above water in a health care sea of increasing complexity. Today, many managers' workloads include responsibilities and accountabilities for managing interdisciplinary staff, facilitating collaborative and evidence-based practice, introducing new models of care, and inspiring research. This edition offers a Management 101 strategy coupled with an urgent call to act sooner rather than later in the name of professional nursing care. The back-to-basics plan works. At least it proves a more useful tool than the continued spinning of wheels of which so many managers complain. I hope this book will inspire you to grab hold of a potential lifeline to pull yourself ashore and create your new beginning by powering up your practice. *The best way to predict your future is to create it.* You can do it. You must.

This edition will provide you with quick access to hard-hitting insights and strategies for a back-to-basics approach to managing professional practice no matter what is happening around you. My hope is that this new edition will add skills to your managerial toolkit that will assist you in leading nurses and other interprofessional staff working in today's complex health care environments to accomplish four goals:

1. To shift your focus to adopt, lead, and facilitate a back-to-basics approach to care that ensures professional nursing practice, quality care outcomes, and quality of work life;
2. To encourage you to boldly spread your professional leadership wings to become a champion of change by facilitating removal of barriers to professional practice;
3. To fearlessly require staff to clearly articulate their professional roles, adhere to their standards of practice, honor their code of ethics as they work together, and, above all, keep the patient at the center of care;
4. To have fun with all of the above.

Barbara Fry

Acknowledgments

In reflecting on the messages in this book, I think back to when, as a 10-year-old, I sat next to my father's aunt Nell Stewart, a sister of Isabel Maitland Stewart, one of the founders of nursing education in the United States. As I listened to her stories of adventures they shared riding horseback through the Rocky Mountains, trips to the Caribbean setting up libraries, and highlights of Isabel's nursing career, the stone was cast. I knew then that I wanted to become a nurse. Isabel's beliefs about nursing have deeply shaped my own. I am forever grateful to the nurses who have also shared their stories, deepened my insight, and fueled my passion for the profession I love. My resolve is never ending to do all that I can to advocate for conditions that allow professional nursing practice to thrive and the quality of patient care to excel.

Thank you, dear Peter, for your continued loving support.

PART

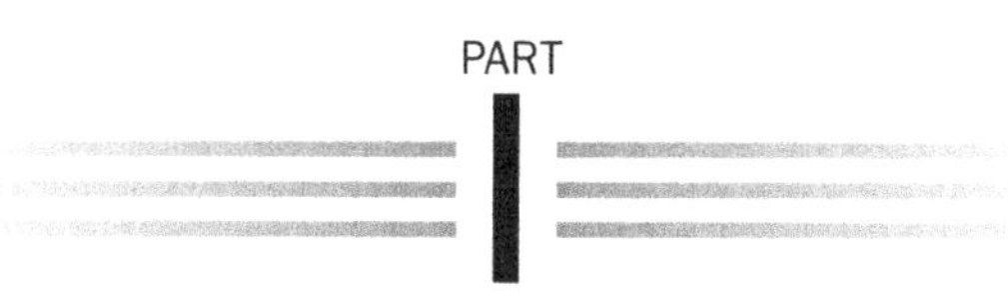

The Bottom Line

Managing What *Now* Lies Beneath

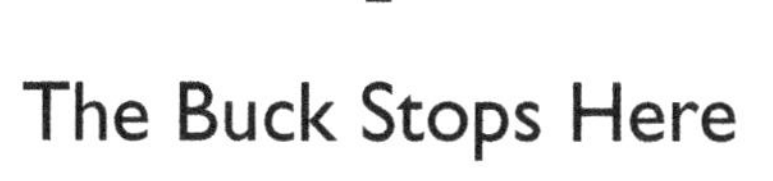

The Buck Stops Here

Managing Professional Practice

This chapter reinforces your ultimate accountability as the nurse manager to ensure that professional nursing practice is alive and well in your workplace. It also serves to remind you that despite the heavy demands of managing day-to-day operations, nurse managers are accountable for managing an interprofessional and diverse staff, while ensuring practice that is collaborative, evidence based, and guided by professional standards of practice and codes of ethics.

In this chapter, you will learn:

1. The nurse manager's accountabilities and responsibilities for leading professional practice environments in a rapidly changing health care system
2. Specific strategies for demonstrating leadership and "walking the talk" about professional practice in the workplace

TOWARD A NEW WAY OF BEING

The role of today's nurse managers is a work in progress that is rapidly evolving within frenetically paced and changing health care environments. Today's nurse managers, in addition to managing the operations of a particular service, are now required to have an organizational and community presence, effectively pulling them away from their geographical area of responsibility. When they are in their clinical areas (sometimes multiple areas), in addition to managing operations, they serve as nursing practice leaders, facilitators, coaches, and traffic cops (spending their time directing any number of individuals coming at them from all directions). In addition, inspiring trust and generating attitudes promoting collaboration and professionalism, they are ever mindful of creating an environment where people want to work (let us not forget many "other related duties," as well). Above all, managers have responsibility for safe, competent, and ethical practice in the provision of nursing care. Added to their workload are managing patient care and family crises, committee participation, and possibly covering another clinical area for a vacationing colleague. Is it any wonder that many nurse managers question their sanity as they try to keep all the balls in the air?

Many nurse managers continue to have little or no formal preparation for this vital role. Most stepped into the role as a temporary replacement, were "promoted" for their clinical excellence, or "volunteered" when no others would step up to the plate. Moreover, most receive little organizational support, and funding seems minimal for professional development of middle management. Owing to the gradual recognition that the nurse manager is the key to clinical excellence this situation is (thankfully) improving. A day in the life of a nurse manager usually means 80% of his or her time is spent managing operational issues and dealing with erratic, unexpected, or unpredictable incidents (hereafter fondly referred to as "brushfire management").

24/7/365 IS NOT ENOUGH TIME

Most nurse managers are ultimately professionally accountable and responsible for the overall quality of care delivered to patients and clients **24 hours a day, 7 days a week, 365 days a year**. However, much of their time is spent away from the practice setting. How do mangers find the time to ensure that professional practice is alive and well within their service area(s)? All too often, many nurse managers reluctantly admit that they do not have enough time to monitor practice because of other demands, are not physically present in their clinical settings long enough to know what is really going on, or confess that it has been a long time (if ever) since they actively promoted the standards in everyday practice. Despite the fact that individual nurses and other health care professionals are accountable and responsible for their individual practice, and the availability of clinical support (if they are lucky) from clinical nurse educators, mentors, and nurse specialists, no one but the nurse manager has the authority or professional accountability to manage nursing practice to ensure that standards of practice are met. With the increasing demand for evidence-based practice, this becomes a significant additional challenge. Bottom line: the buck stops with the nurse manager who is ultimately responsible for the overall delivery of quality nursing care. Managers must know and never assume that what is going on at the bedside is delivered by the right person, at the right time, and in the right way according to the care provider's scope of practice, standards, and code of ethics.

MANAGING CHANGE TO ENSURE SAFE, COMPETENT, ETHICAL PRACTICE

When significant organizational change challenges the practice environment individuals and teams react. How well they navigate change depends on many factors, including the leadership and culture of the unit or service and the broader organization. Professional caring behavior can be influenced positively or negatively by variables that include past experience with change, quality of communication during the change process, workload, physical and psychological well-being of individual staff members, attitudes of other staff members, professional autonomy, and nursing leadership.

In situations where change is managed well, staff is inclined to thrive despite the challenges when professionalism and excellence in care provision become the goals of the practice environment and staff members are led and inspired by a strong nurse manager.

When change is not managed well staff feels disconnected, powerless, disrespected, and anxious about their future. This uncertainty and anxiety may lead to physical, emotional, and psychological strain causing staff to retreat into survival mode. In an environment that seems to be spinning out of control, with ever increasing burdens of rising acuity levels, task-focused care, lack of time, and inadequate staffing, nurses draw upon their energy reserves and vigorously focus on the tasks related to getting the job done. The risk is great of focusing exclusively on the tasks and technical aspects of nursing practice, and believing that "there isn't time for that other touchy-feely stuff." But when nurses do this they place their professional practice in jeopardy, falling well short of their scope of practice by losing sight of the nursing process outlined in the legislation and standards and upon which their license depends.

When nursing and staff practice falls short of professional requirements it is essential that nurse managers not delay in dealing with the situation. Coincidentally, this is usually the time when nurse managers and staff complain about "absent leadership." Redressing this situation is no easy task for a manager. More than ever nurse managers must be available to make their way back to the bedside or practice setting if for no other reason than to ensure that patient/client care and safety are in no way compromised because of a failure to uphold the standards of practice.

PROFESSIONAL PRACTICE STANDARDS CHECK-IN

How familiar are you, currently, with the standards of practice for nursing and the code of ethics for staff and nursing leadership? While many nurse managers have a tacit understanding of these professional practice guidelines some will readily admit that they do not significantly factor into their daily stream of consciousness. If that is the case, then this must change. **Regardless of the demands that are placed on you during organizational change, your commitment to maintaining nursing practice and quality care outcomes according to the standards and code must remain stalwart and at the forefront.**

To do this, you must first give yourself time to reflect on your own familiarity with the standards; how you use the standards to guide your administrative practice; and the degree to which you model the standards among your staff on a day-to-day basis. It might also be helpful to answer the following questions:

- To what degree do the standards of practice and the code of ethics influence our professional practice environment?
- In what ways do all staff members demonstrate evidence of utilization of the standards of practice in their everyday practice and therapeutic relationships with patients and clients?
- How do staff members treat one another professionally, and in what way do they apply the standards to their collegial and professional relationships?
- In what ways do the standards of practice influence patient/client care communication?
- How much do the standards factor into creating a respectful workplace and healthy workplace relationships?
- How much time each day do you allocate to discussing patient care and nursing practice and linking them to the standards of practice?

PRACTICE STANDARDS IN A PRACTICE SETTING

When standards of practice significantly influence a practice setting:

- Leading and managing nursing staff will require you at all times to hold staff accountable and responsible for the provision of safe, competent, and ethical nursing practice according to their standards of practice.
- All nursing staff will incorporate both technical and interpersonal aspects of practice in their care. Professional nursing practice requires a high level of scientific knowledge, hands-on competencies, and relational skills in the provision of comprehensive care. Although nurses in some practice settings, such as an intensive care unit or emergency department, must focus on the technical aspects of care whereas others, such as psychiatric/mental health nurses, may be more focused on the therapeutic interpersonal relationship, all nurses must demonstrate both aspects of care in their daily practice in each interaction with their client/patient. Focusing exclusively on one aspect

denies patients and clients the full benefits of nursing's scope of practice.

- Nurses will adhere to and routinely reference their nursing standards of practice and code of ethics in their delivery of care.
- Nurse managers will ensure other interprofessional staff members meet their professional codes of ethics and standards of practice when working in their area of clinical practice.
- Nurse managers will ensure their personal adherence to the standards of practice for all registered nurses as well as those for nurse leaders (if they are identified).
- The nurse manager's scope of practice, influence, and communication will extend beyond the physical boundaries of his or her clinical practice setting to include the organization, the community, and beyond.
- Nurse managers will spend regular time in their practice settings communicating face to face with staff to monitor practice, ensure staff have the necessary tools to do their work, and build trust and support.
- Staff members will expect nurse managers to do what they say they will do.
- Nurse managers will regularly demonstrate coaching, mentoring, and support for staff's professional development.
- Nurse managers will successfully manage change.

The nurse manager must occasionally remind nursing staff that their foremost purpose is to serve their patients. Especially during times of rapid change, it is sometimes difficult for staff members to keep their eyes on the ball. Once in a while it is helpful to be reminded to step back, breathe, and refocus.

STRATEGIES FOR PROMOTING STANDARDS OF PRACTICE

Clearly Communicate Your Expectations

- First ask staff what they believe is your role followed by their expectations of your leadership.
- Tell staff about your managerial/operational and professional role accountabilities—that staff members must meet their professional and organizational standards of care; ensure the provision of safe,

competent, and ethical care to achieve quality patient outcomes; support professional practice by providing necessary resources for staff to perform their roles; manage the budget; and create a place where staff want to work. That's pretty much it in a nutshell!

- Identify six key points about your expectations for a professional nursing practice environment, such as respect, transparent communication, collaboration, accountability, compassion, and healthy workplace relationships. Provide each staff member with a hard copy of the points.
- Ask staff to respond to what you said: what they liked; what they did not understand, and any other thoughts they might have.
- At least once a year schedule a review of the standards of practice and code of ethics.
- Pick one or two standards and begin a conversation, for example, about what accountability in professional nursing practice looks like to patients, peers, and other team members.
- Tell staff you plan to spend some time with each of them at some point to discuss their practice, which will include a discussion about nursing plans of care, how standards influence their practice, and their evidence to support nursing interventions. (This is a key exercise to assess staff's level of knowledge about theory and practice, and identify where the "hot spots" are for learning and possibilities).

Other Activities to Reinforce Professional Practice Standards

- In nursing rounds, periodically discuss which standard(s) influenced care decision making.
- Invite a clinical nurse specialist, nurse educator, or practitioner to conduct regularly scheduled lunch-and-learn sessions that focus on practice standards and research in nursing practice.
- Discuss with other nurse managers how they use the standards to reinforce professional practice.

THE BOTTOM LINE IS NOT ABOUT MONEY

Nurse managers can easily be consumed by directing most of their professional energies toward managing the operational aspects of a busy practice setting. There are never enough hours in the day. But when you step back and, with a critical eye, examine the underlying engine that drives the practice setting much is revealed. What you may see is very busy people trying to do the best they can for the patients/clients they serve. But you will also see that much of the operational approach is related to entrenched patterns of thinking and behaving (i.e., "This is the way we always do things around here"), the informal culture, or reactive practice in response to the bone-breaking pressure of a system under siege. In the background lie the all too easily forgotten guidelines of professional practice that are at risk of extinction in the consciousness of practitioners.

As the nurse manager, your job first and foremost is to ensure that excellent quality nursing care is delivered according to the standards of practice and code of ethics. Your second job is to manage the resources for nurses and other clinicians to do their jobs.

FAST FACTS in a NUTSHELL

- Nurse managers are accountable and responsible 24/7/365 for the quality of nursing care delivered in their clinical practice setting.
- Nurse managers must deal with nursing practices that are inconsistent with the professional standards of practice and the code of ethics.

2

Power, Politics, and Possibilities

Managing the Art of the Possible

Savvy nurse managers know the importance of becoming comfortable with the "P" words: positive personal and professional power, becoming political, and seeing the possibilities in a changing workplace. The more nurse managers know and use these words to guide their leadership actions, the more influential and successful they will become in facilitating the critical linkages among professional nursing practice, quality of work life, and organizational success.

In this chapter, you will learn:

1. Attitude is the seat of personal and professional power
2. How "P" words can transform your professional practice and that of your staff
3. Strategies to guide your political development using personal and professional power

"P" WORDS: POSITIVE POWER, POLITICS, AND POSSIBILITIES

In the early days of health care restructuring, the battle cry of "lead, follow, or get out of the way" heralded a paradigm shift that resulted in organizational restructuring, revision of work processes, and reallocation of resources. Nurse managers were also challenged to manage their budgets "or we will find someone who will." In the end, they were left feeling they had few choices. While some bravely decided to lead despite being unsure about what this new leadership would look like, many fell victim to an overwhelming sense of powerlessness. Hoping to defend themselves against job loss, nurse managers dug into their workplace bunkers, struggled to support their anxiety-ridden staff members, and turned most of their attention inward in survival mode. They focused on their budgets, doing more with less, and maintaining the status quo for fear of making a career-limiting move.

POWER, POLITICS, AND POSSIBILITY PONDERABLES

Today even with positional power, many nurse managers continue to feel powerlessness, caught in the middle, and that they have the responsibility without the authority. It is important to try to determine how much power you have in the organization by considering the following:

- How much personal and professional power do you have to influence staff, your peer group, and the organization?
- How effective is your interpersonal communication and ability to speak up about barriers to professional practice or practice issues in your clinical environment?
- How comfortable are you in sharing power through delegation and collaboration?
- Are you politically savvy enough to know what is happening beyond the four walls of your unit or organization; to acquire the resources you need to provide safe, ethical, and competent care; and to manage complex workplace relationships?
- What grade would you receive on a nurse manager report card if one existed?
- And, by the way, what is your "possibility quotient"? That is, how excited are you about the possibilities that exist in the evolving world of health care? Do you see your situation as a crisis or an opportunity?

The nursing literature tells us that nurses tend to shy away from the use of "P" words, especially *power* and *politics*. Power is regarded as antithetical to caring. Nurses will substitute *empower* for the word *power* to soften the perception of what may sound offensive to caring ears. And while nurses can readily express their feelings of powerlessness, they struggle with conversations about developing a sense of personal and professional power.

Nurse managers can model the use of positive language that reflects personal and professional power in order to help staff members move beyond using "soft" language that demeans, minimizes, or marginalizes their practice. The manager is the person with the positional power to lead nurses to discover the possibilities that lie within and the capacity to help facilitate their professional transformation.

FAST FACTS in a NUTSHELL

- Nurses must get comfortable with "P" words.
- These include personal and professional power, politics, and possibilities.
- Using "P" words to create new conversations can lead to new learning, growing, and changing.

POWER TO CHOOSE YOUR ATTITUDE

Before you can adequately lead your staff in getting comfortable with personal and professional power, politics, and possibilities in a changing workplace you must first determine where you fit. To do this, **give yourself the gift of time to reflect on your own quality of life at work, your attitude, and your willingness to change.** Ask yourself the following questions:

- Am I excited about the future? Or am I scared to death that I cannot do what is expected of me?
- Given the options of "lead, follow or get out of the way," what will I choose?
- Do I have the courage to change?

ATTITUDE MATTERS

The following statements can serve as guiding principles for you to embrace as you consider the scope of your personal and professional power as a nurse manager:

1. **The one thing I have power over in my work life is the attitude I choose in response to change.**
2. No one or no situation is responsible for my attitude. I choose my attitude.
3. The quality of my work life future and workplace relationships will largely depend on the attitude I choose.
4. I know that the best way to predict my future is to create it.
5. The only person I can change is me.
6. To successfully manage my changing role and workplace, I must be willing to learn, grow, and change.
7. Memo to self: For every crisis there is opportunity, there are two sides to every coin, yada, yada, yada!

CHOOSING POWERLESSNESS

What attitude will you choose? If you choose powerlessness:

- You will quickly learn that your behavior will lead to acting powerless.
- You will talk like a victim by whining about almost everything, wondering why others don't understand "how difficult it is for us . . . ," or complaining that, "I don't know what's going on around here, nobody tells us anything."
- **You may unwittingly give permission to your staff to become victims as well.** In organizational speak, this is known as the cascade effect, in which behaviors at the top of the organization spillover and get played out in the actions of the frontline staff.

FAST FACTS in a NUTSHELL

- You have power to choose your attitude. (The Devil doesn't make you do it!)
- Attitude is a powerful determinant in quality of work life.
- There are positives and negatives in every situation; the key is to find and act on the positives.

CHOOSING A POSITIVE PERSONAL AND PROFESSIONAL WAY OF BEING

As the nurse manager, you can be the most positive influence on the staff's ability to adapt to a changing workplace. **When you choose a positive attitude as a personal and professional way of being, you become personally and professionally powerful.** You will not only strengthen your own sense of well-being, you will inspire others to do the same.

12 TERRIFIC STRATEGIES FOR POWERING UP PERSONALLY AND PROFESSIONALLY

1. Create "a-ha" moments for yourself by reflecting on and admitting that in today's complex health care environments you cannot be all things to all people; that you do not have all the answers; that you will do the best possible job within the limitations of your human, fiscal, and personal resources—and that the world will keep on turning. To that end, try the 11 strategies that follow.
2. **Resolve to embark on a journey of new learning to increase your personal and professional power for leading change in the workplace.** Think about traveling along a metaphorical road that has many side roads. Some you will take, others you may not choose. A few may entice you halfway along on your journey, others may come to a dead end. (When that happens, simply turn round and choose another path.) As Yogi Berra said, "When you come to a fork in the road, take it!"
3. Recognize that this journey is not one more thing you must do. Make it an adventure in self-discovery, and [*gasp*] it might even be fun!
4. Reflect upon someone you once worked with or currently work with —someone you consider to possess exemplary leadership qualities. What inspires you about them? Write down their amazing qualities and think about your own style of managing and leading.
5. Consider the following: What are your strengths? What areas could you improve on? How closely aligned are your qualities with those of the person you most admire?

6. Identify the relationships and situations in the workplace that push your "powerless" buttons.
7. List situations over which you have no control and immediately put them aside.
8. Create a priority list for dealing with situations over which you have influence and control. Name the issues and create an action plan.
9. Learn everything you can about managing the power dynamics and relationships across the levels in the organization.
10. Develop a personal learning plan for building on your leadership competencies that will assist you in your journey toward a new way of being.
11. Give yourself permission to try on new behaviors to see what fits. At first this may feel uncomfortable to you and to others but stick with it and remind yourself that you cannot be responsible for how others react toward you the emerging new you!
12. Lighten up, be kind to yourself, and don't forget to have fun.

POWERING UP POLITICALLY

Political acumen is necessary for nurse managers to secure resources, manage conflict, and build relationships to get the work done and ensure optimum levels of care. Consider these political skills ponderables:

- How skillful are you in inspiring others?
- How well do you engage your staff and influence colleagues in considering new possibilities, directions, and policies?
- How in tune are you with your staff's power dynamics—that is, registered nurses (RNs), licensed practical/vocational nurses (LPNs/LVNs), and other members of the interdisciplinary team?
- How well informed are you about the power dynamics within your organization?
- How well do you interface with other nonnursing managers and leaders?
- How good are you at breaking through the organizational "silos" and forging new relationships?
- How well do you manage conflict?

FAST FACTS in a NUTSHELL

- Women are inherently relational, which makes them well suited for the political arena.
- Essential to nursing practice is the professional management of relationships, and nurses are well educated for political arena. They just don't necessarily recognize or name their interactions as such.

By turning these ponderables into action steps for new learning you are well on your journey toward effective management of your changing workplace.

A NOTE OF CAUTION: WHEN NURSE MANAGERS "HANG OUT" WITH STAFF

The power dynamics between nurse managers and staff is a delicate one. When nurse managers party with staff and socialize with staff on a regular basis, mixed messages are sent. Because the incumbent nurse manager is required to manage performance, evaluate quality of service, and hire and fire, socializing can lead to blurred professional and social boundaries. When a manager's friendship is tossed into the professional relationship mix, the resulting situation has the potential to create relational hardship, workplace tension, accusations of favoritism and unfairness, ambivalence, and uncertainty. "Hanging out" with staff becomes particularly problematic when the manager has to discipline a staff member who is also a good friend.

There are many reasons why this dynamic develops, but it is usually explained as a means for nurse managers to "get staff to like them" or to prove to staff that they, too, are "real nurses." Another reason could be the manager's attempt to reinforce the concept of team, the idea that "we're all in this together." While these strategies may seem to work in the short term, they rarely work in the long term. **Bottom line: You cannot be a friend and effectively manage staff.** In a professional practice environment, relationships must be grounded in professional behavior for both managers and staff. In locations where "everybody knows everybody," particularly in small communities, it is very important to have the conversation with staff about boundaries around professional relationships and how they are to be managed in the workplace.

FAST FACTS in a NUTSHELL

- Bottom line: You cannot be a friend and effectively manage staff.

MANAGING THE ART OF THE POSSIBLE

In a changing workplace, nurse managers know that curve balls can be thrown at anytime from anywhere! Plans and people come and go and the only constant is change. Our world of work in health care is an ever changing reality. To paraphrase Albert Einstein, we cannot solve today's problems with yesterday's solutions. We have to find new ways of working together, and no template exists to show us how to move forward. To that end there are only possibilities. Nurse managers and staff must step away from self-limiting comments such as "We've always done it this way." Instead, ask the question, "What is possible or what possibilities exist?" These types of questions throw the doors wide open to new ways of thinking, working, and being.

Simply asking about possibilities inspires new conversations and stimulates new learning opportunities to facilitate a journey on the path of change. Nurse managers have the power to facilitate self-discovery in each staff member to inspire the professional power that lies within the staff group. Transformed nursing staff is capable of exceeding performance expectations, creating an environment where people want to work, and demonstrating personal and professional power in their practice. Staff energy is palpable and the possibilities are endless.

Summary

- "P" words such as positive personal and professional power in practice, politics, and possibility can be the foundation for individual and workplace transformation.
- Facilitating professional power through self-discovery and self-mastery is both a gift and a responsibility of nurse managers.

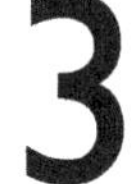

Competencies for a Changing Workplace

Managing New Rules, New Roles

Do your staff members cling to old patterns of working just because "we've always done it this way"? This chapter will assist you in facilitating their understanding of the need for all of us to acquire the competencies that help in adapting to a new workplace environment. As new rules, roles, and competencies emerge, each of us must make a choice—to move toward a new way of being, remain the same, or stick our heads in the sand. Will this situation precipitate a personal crisis or professional opportunity? The choice is ours to make!

In this chapter, you will learn:

1. The impact of transitioning from the "good ol' days" to a new way of being
2. The key competencies that will positively influence nursing practice in a changing workplace
3. Strategies to manage the new competencies

OH, THE TIMES THEY ARE A CHANGIN'

Reinforcing reality is a principle we all learned in psychiatric and mental health nursing. It remains a useful tool for today's nurse managers in helping staff understand the requirement for personal and professional change in in order to thrive in today's practice settings. It is fair to say that many organizational changes are driven by the forces of global economics and technological advancements. Thus, they are beyond staff control. However, some staff members undoubtedly believe that all this change is the direct result of some the hare-brained scheme developed by unknown people sitting in a dark room deliberately planning ways to mess up their lives.

REMEMBERING THE GOOD OL' DAYS

In the past, changes in nursing practice often resulted from internal requirements to improve patient care efficiencies, quality of care, and service delivery. Today, care provision is complex, being subjected to the influence of budgets, technology, acuity levels, changing demographics, intergenerational and culturally diverse workforces, dwindling human resources, and restructuring. In a world where change is the only constant, **nurses must embrace new competencies, new rules, new roles, new structures, and new opportunities** whether they like it or not! Your job is to help them understand and manage these requirements.

EXTRA! EXTRA! READ ALL ABOUT IT! PROFESSIONAL NURSING PRACTICE IN A STATE OF TRANSITION

Many organizations and professional disciplines are finding themselves caught in the middle of a clash of the Ages (as in historical eras) and often, ages (as in younger versus older staff) as workplaces evolve from the hierarchical mindset and practices of the Industrial Age to the Age of Information and Technology and then to the Age of Creativity. Quite a leap in a matter of a few decades!

Transitioning and adapting to a changing workplace can be particularly challenging for staff who are seniors (born before

1945) and their baby boomer colleagues (born before 1965) who spent the majority of their work lives in highly structured, top-down, command-and-control environments.

YOU'VE COME A LONG WAY, BABY!

The role of the nurse manager, formerly known as the head nurse, has undergone unprecedented changes over the past three decades that include changes in title, scope of leadership practice, and place within the organization. Some nurses argue that these changes and expectations have made things worse. Others can barely contain their excitement about the opportunities that come with a position that has the authority to directly influence and bring improvements in the quality of care outcomes, service delivery, nursing practice, and the direction of the organization. The following discussion provides a brief, tongue-in-cheek glimpse at the role of the head nurse in the near past (the sixties, seventies, eighties, and nineties) and concludes with an overview of the ever-evolving role of nurse/clinical/health services manager.

A BIRD'S-EYE VIEW OF THE GOOD OL' DAYS OF NURSING MANAGEMENT

Many nurses gaze fondly on the past, longing for the stability and perceived desirability of seemingly less complex times when the "head nurse" was always there, answered all questions related to patient care, ruled her (for the nurse was almost always female) roost with an authoritarian style of leadership, and assumed all accountability for patient care outcomes, leaving many staff nurses feeling largely unaccountable for the outcomes of their practice. Head nurses were *the* source, the "go-to" person, and the solution for all things nursing. They had little influence or presence in organizational decision making, their operations and budgets were decentralized to those who had little or no knowledge of the practice setting, and hiring of their staff was a function of human resources.

That's Not My Job!

In the not-so-distant past, the head nurse's influence extended only as far as the job descriptions of staff allowed. These descriptions were prescriptive and numbered, with a final category of "other related duties" tacked on the end. They frequently became a bone of contention between union and management. If staff members were asked to do something not listed in their job descriptions, the response was likely to be, "That's not in my job description, if you make me do it, I'll grieve!" In the good ol' days, the union would be all over the head nurse like fleas on a dog. The head nurse was silenced.

The Workplace How-To Policy and Procedure Manual: Instrument of the Devil?

More than almost anything else in those years, policy and procedure manuals influenced practice. Originally designed to guide safe practice, the manuals soon morphed into a bureaucratic monster that covered every imaginable action staff might ever have to take. Best practice guidelines did not exist. Once dutifully written—their completion heralded, read, and initialled by staff—"P & P's," as they were fondly termed, were quickly banished to ever-expanding bookshelves until called forth to duty as the final pronouncement of what must happen next! Taking on mythic proportions they quickly became the showcased and dust-covered tomes that many considered to be the "law" in nursing practice. If staff members were asked to perform a task or procedure that could not be found in the policy and procedure manual, they might be overheard saying, "If it isn't written in the P & P manual, it doesn't exist, and I won't or can't do that!"

The Union–Management Hard Line

In the past, relationships between union and management were more adversarial and inclined to focus less on professional practice and more on wages and job preservation. The workforce was primarily homogenous with respect to gender, ethnicity, and age.

TODAY'S NURSE MANAGERS

Today's nurse managers work in what Vaill (1996), aptly refers to as "white water" workplace environments, where they frequently have operational responsibility for complex and multiple practice settings and 24-hour, 365-day accountability for the delivery of safe, ethical, and competent nursing and clinical care. In addition, many are involved at the organizational and community levels, participate in special interest groups, and are researchers and presenters at national and international conferences.

Bye-Bye Job Descriptions?

Written job descriptions cannot possibly cover every aspect of nursing's full scope of practice. Rapid technological changes, delegated medical acts, and changing patient demographics make it difficult to keep job descriptions current. Because of the complexities of the practice environment and patient acuity, staff must be flexible and do whatever it takes within the bounds of their scopes of practice to safely, ethically, and competently care for patients and clients.

Policy and Procedure Manuals: Relics of the Past?

Nursing staff's overreliance on policy and procedure manuals must slowly go the way of dinosaurs and be replaced by technological resources, critical thinking skills of practitioners, and evidence-based practice. Because Generation Xers and Ys prefer to use technology-based resources rather than reading manuals, and want to help the environment by "saving the trees," they may add momentum to the urgent need for ready access to information and on-line technology. The introduction of technology into the workplace, especially handheld devices, has become a large problem in almost all practice environments. It can enhance practice with rapid access to information on best practice or it can be a source of great angst among managers and patients within the context of social media. For some staff the handheld device has become a lifeline attached to a body part; one that they must regularly check to avoid withdrawal setting in!

Nurse Managers and Unions: Adversaries or Collaborators?

The health care workplace today is all about relationships. Adversarial relationships between unions and management are no longer productive in moving the profession forward. While many staff from the senior and boomer generations were influenced by, and benefited from the demands of unions (for better workplace conditions and pay), younger generations are less inclined to feel the need for outside organizational support in these areas. Responding to this demographic shift, **progressive union and nursing management relationships today are focused less on demands for job security and pay incentives and more on professional development and learning opportunities** aimed at improving quality of work life, healthy workplace relationships, professionalism, and improved care practices.

FAST FACTS in a NUTSHELL

- What is hot? New competencies: risk taking, creativity, flexibility, and innovation.
- What is not? Rigid job descriptions, policy and procedure manuals, and command-and-control leadership styles.
- What's exciting? Collaborative union–management relationships.

NEW COMPETENCIES: RISK TAKING, INNOVATION, CREATIVITY, AND FLEXIBILITY

To lead and manage today's nursing staff, nurse managers can facilitate staff members' consideration of how they can enhance their practice and professional presence by strengthening, incorporating, and reenforcing "new" competencies that enable them to thrive in a changing practice environment. But, here's the rub. **These competencies are not new for nurses.** They are already deeply embedded in nursing practice although not usually named as such. Rarely do nurses refer to themselves as *innovators* (knowledge workers), *risk takers*, *creative*, or *flexible*. They are more likely to say, "I am just a nurse" or "I am here to help you."

Risk Taking

Risk taking within the context of clinical practice is not about putting patients at risk. It is about a willingness to change, try something new, offer to lead when others refuse, and speak out when others choose silence. It is also about stretching beyond our comfort zones and occasionally taking a leap of faith. For example, risk taking occurs when nurse managers challenge the status quo by speaking out against organizational barriers to professional nursing practice.

Innovation

The word *innovation* is relatively new as a description of nursing actions in daily clinical practice. Nurses have always been innovators but often prefer to keep that a secret (remember the torn sheets used to create breast binders when supplies ran out?). Typically nurses do not think of or identify their practice as innovative. Instead, they diminish or dismiss their actions through comments such as, "I just did what I had to do for the well-being of my patient." Nurses must speak up about their innovations in practice and share them beyond the confines of their immediate workplace. Managers can help nurses reframe their actions as innovative rather than "just routine." When you do so, observe the shift in their nonverbal response and how they now perceive themselves: Fascinating!

Creativity

In the Industrial Age mindset, the word *creativity* was not a normal part of the organizational lexicon in nursing. In fact, policies, procedures, and practices were designed to create conformity in an era when creative thinkers were often labeled as "off the wall," "boat rockers," and worse. Staff members are now asked to become creative by "thinking out of the box." However, many seniors and boomers, scarred by organizational change and haunted by memories of recrimination and putdowns, believe that it is not safe to speak out for fear of once again being labeled, marginalized, or put at risk by making a career-limiting move. Creativity can only flourish in a workplace where mistakes are considered opportunities to learn, inquiry is valued, trust is high, mutual respect is expected, and high value is placed on knowledge gleaned from creative thought as opposed to habit.

Flexibility

Flexibility in assignments, tasks, as well as participation in learning opportunities and processes, can inspire flexibility among nursing staff, strengthen interpersonal relationships, and boost morale. Flexibility in practice settings requires us to do whatever it takes to meet the complex needs of our patients/clients and support the interprofessional team and relationships. It is no longer acceptable in practice to snarl, "That's not my job!" Workplaces steeped in informal rules and insistence on conformity to do things according to "the way we do things around here," stunt personal and professional growth, and deny patients the full benefits of best practice and nurses working to full scope. A "can-do" attitude among staff promotes patient-centered care and demonstrates an energy and willingness to learn, grow, and change.

FAST FACTS in a NUTSHELL

- The new competencies are risk taking, innovation, creativity, and flexibility.
- These "new" competencies are not new to nurses. They have always been integral to nursing practice; we just never named them as such.

FROM NO NAME TO NEW NAME: TIPS TO HELP STAFF REFRAME THEIR PRACTICE

Nurse managers can inspire staff to build a thriving workplace culture by using contemporary language to reflect nursing practice. It may feel awkward at first but will eventually become mainstream. Try the following:

- Change the language; change the culture. Try incorporating words such as *relational, respectful, innovative, spirit, honor, research*, and *innovative practice*. Frequently linking statements to the literature is also helpful in shifting the cultural dialogue. Instead of saying, "Jane had a good idea," try saying, "Jane was very creative . . . " Or, rather than "Susie volunteered . . . " try, "Susie demonstrated leadership when she . . . "

- Help staff members reframe their work. Replace "I'm just a nurse so I don't know . . . ," try, "As a registered or licensed practical nurse, the research tells me that . . . "
- Talk about collaboration when you talk about "working together."
- The word *team* has been overworked to the point where staff members' eyes glaze over at its very mention. Try words like *workgroup, peers, staff group,* and *colleagues.*
- Try to avoid saying, "**My staff.**" This removes your relationship from a professional context to personal ownership and conveys a "power over" dynamic.
- Teach staff members to avoid using the word *girls* when they refer to their professional relationships (apologies to male staff members). Refer to staff as *staff* or *team* or *colleague* or use their first and last name.
- Identify other words that subtly diminish the value of nurses and professional practice in the workplace, such as "just did this."
- Incorporate language that profiles nurses as knowledge workers. Use phrases such as, "According to the literature" or "The evidence suggests . . . "
- You go first. Be the first in your organization to model professional nursing practice "speak."
- Watch your body language. Ensure that your words and tone match what your body is communicating, for instance, when standing with arms crossed in front (resistance), scowling (displeased), or smiling (pleased). This level of self-awareness is vital to your nurse manager repertoire!

FAST FACTS in a NUTSHELL

Summary

- If you want to change the culture of your practice setting, try language that reflects a new way of being and revitalize your nursing culture by incorporating words such as *relational, respectful, innovative, spirit, honor, research,* and *literature.* You will be amazed how quickly this catches on in changing behaviors and inspire confidence in your leadership!

REFERENCE

Vaill, P. (1996). *Learning as a way of being: Strategies for survival in a world of permanent white water.* San Francisco, CA: Jossey-Bass.

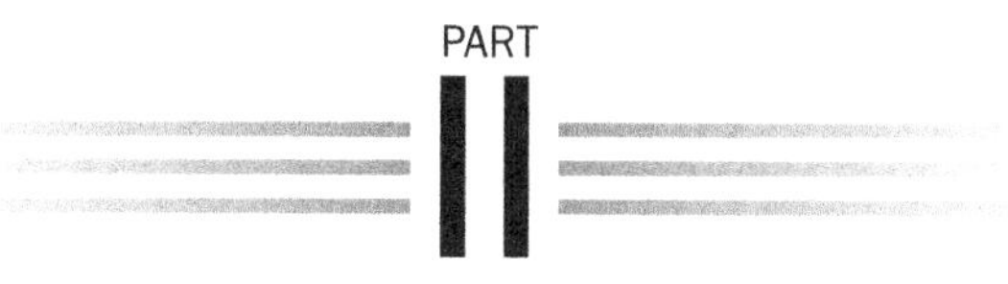

The Here and Now

Managing New Realities

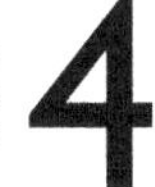

4 Anticipating Change

Managing Staff Anxiety, Uncertainty, and Fear

Change is the only constant in health care organizations as they adapt to today's realities. Staff nurses face countless challenges as they struggle to provide care in environments fraught with uncertainty and unrelenting pressures. Simply anticipating the next round of changes can set off, throughout their practice settings, an undercurrent of staff anxiety and fear. Many staff members turn to their nurse manager, looking for answers to questions when there may be none. Left unexpressed, fear-based emotions and behaviors can spread like a malignancy, taking on a life of their own that has a negative impact on quality of work life and patient care. This chapter will help you to manage and lead staff through that tangle of fear, anxiety, and uncertainty about their future.

In this chapter, you will learn:

1. The importance of identifying, within yourself and staff, change-induced anxiety and fear of the unknown
2. Strategies for managing anxiety and fear in the workplace

ANXIETY, UNCERTAINTY, AND FEAR IN A CHANGING WORKPLACE

Anxiety and fear in a workplace shrouded in a climate of uncertainty are heightened during significant organizational change. The constant fear of job loss poses the greatest threat to the emotional well-being of most leaders and staff. At such a time nurse managers bear several burdens. In addition to managing the operational aspects of a practice setting, **nurse managers must be adept at identifying and helping themselves and staff members manage emotional, psychological, and behavioral responses to change.**

When organizational change requires cost cutting and new efficiency measures, nurse managers are under extraordinary pressure to do more with less particularly when their overall performance is being judged on whether they achieve the bottom line. Often caught between the proverbial rock and a hard place, they too may fall victim to anxiety, uncertainty, fear, and feelings of self-doubt. Many may wonder, "How do I support my staff when I am feeling so vulnerable?" If you are feeling this way, you need to recognize and acknowledge it. Otherwise you cannot effectively help staff manage their responses. You must take time to reflect on your workplace situation, name what is happening within you, and plan how you will manage.

FAST FACTS in a NUTSHELL

- Many nurse managers and their staff may have to unlearn certain previous coping behaviors and learn new ones to adapt to a changing workplace.
- Nurse managers must go first in modeling a new way of being!

GO AHEAD: EXPRESS YOURSELF!

When faced with anything new it is normal to experience a psychological response ranging from mild apprehension to fear of the unknown, indifference or even excitement. However, when butterflies take up permanent residence in your stomach, fear at work prevents you from doing your job well, and workplace woes spill over to negatively affect your private life, you must first take action to deal with these powerful emotions. When you finally "get a grip" (or "suck it up," to use the present-day vernacular), staff members are more likely to follow your lead and model your fearless behaviors.

Naming our feelings can be difficult for nurses because most of us were taught not to express our feelings while providing patient care (or risk being considered "unprofessional"). Now that the "soft" or people issues are recognized as powerful indicators of organizational success, **nurses must unlearn the imposed stoicism of such dictates as, "Never express your feelings in front of a patient or at work."** Many nurses will face a learning curve as they begin to express (at least to themselves) what they are feeling, name the emotion, and deal with it. Some nurses have adopted this new behavior and verbalize all too well. When nurses whine, natter, and complain in front of patients, they have crossed a professional boundary into a danger zone where they can transfer their fear onto the patient. Add this problem to your "To-Do" list and address it ASAP.

Both large-scale and small-scale organizational change evokes a variety of responses among staff. These **responses range from indifference to the ripple of mild concern and the outright devastation of a tsunami!** The extent of anxiety and fear that exists among staff in your workplace will depend on a number of variables, including:

- The magnitude of change (e.g., unit closure, relocation, or the presence of a new nurse manager).
- The organizational and workplace culture.
- How well the organization handled change in the past.
- What change means to individuals (among leaders, frontline staff, and physicians) and their personal circumstances.
- The individual and the staff group's capacity to cope.
- The quality of communication sent out from senior leadership and their nurse manager, and how it is received.

FAST FACTS in a NUTSHELL

- The emotional impact of organizational change can be made better or worse by the nurse manager's ability to communicate clearly, listen carefully, "read" staff accurately, and respond sensitively to staff's needs.
- Listening and responding to what staff members are not saying is vitally important.

THEY NEED TO JUST GET ON WITH IT, RIGHT?

Some senior leaders and nurse managers believe that when changes are required of staff, "they should just get on with it." Lessons learned from the days of reengineering and restructuring tell us that **if we do not attend to the emotional needs of staff, the bottom line will never be achieved.** When needs remain unmet they turn into a cadre of behaviors including anger, frustration, sabotage, and disengagement. While a "stiff upper lip" approach may work for some staff in the short term, in all probability it will lead to emotions being rerouted underground only to surface in behaviors that may lead to poor quality of care, low morale, and increasing use of sick time.

THE IMPORTANCE OF FILLING IN THE BLANKS

In situations where staff members do not understand the need for change or feel unheard when they ask questions, the conditions become ripe for misinformation. **If staff members meet with silence or receive an inadequate or dismissive response to a question, they will fill in the blanks with an answer of their own.** This attempt to plug the communication gap primes the pump for the rumor mill wheel to start churning out the grist for rumors, hearsay, and mayhem!

YOU CAN'T MAKE STAFF BUY INTO CHANGE

During significant organizational change, it is important for nurse managers to know that no matter what the party line or reason given for a specific change—such as, "This change will create a seamless continuum of care for our patients"—the questions on the minds of most staff members will likely be, "What's in it for me? How will this change mess up my life? Will this change really make a difference?" **Generally, staff members will keep these questions to themselves and dutifully nod at the leader's pronouncement.** Leaders look out at the sea of bobbleheads convinced that they have "staff buy-in." They could not be further from the truth. When organizational trust is at an all-time low, leaders need to think about the level of trust in their organization before they can expect staff to endorse proposed changes.

IT'S A MATTER OF TRUST

The worst thing any leader can say to staff with respect to change is, "Trust me, this will result in significant improvement in. . . ." The second worst thing is to say, "We need your buy-in." When you ask staff to buy into change or when you are directed to "get their buy-in" you unwittingly set up a dialogue of resistance in staff member's heads. *Buy in* implies that someone may be trying to get you to do something you might not want to do. It is reminiscent of a conversation you might have with a car salesperson who wants you to buy a wreck! **Buying in is not the issue; trust is.**

FAST FACTS in a NUTSHELL

- Staff members are more likely to engage in change when they can have timely and accurate information, open conversations, feel heard, and trust the messenger.

Even in areas not directly affected by change, most staff members do not trust leader's reassurance that things will be okay, that they will be safe or unaffected by change. Many will experience deep fear or anxiety. Their lack of trust in relation to possible job loss is usually reflected in the statement, "If it can happen to them (others who have lost their jobs), it could happen to us." Nurse managers can help staff manage this fear and bridge the trust gap.

Building organizational and leadership trust is a slow and complex process in which actions speak louder than words. Staff members are generally more willing to trust the nurse manager as a reliable source of information until something happens to break that trust. When nurses trust their manager, they feel comfortable in expressing their opinions, feel heard and respected, and are more willing to listen to feedback about their performance and go where they are led.

When staff members truly "get the reason" for a particular change, they are more likely to engage in activities that support the change initiatives, become involved in implementation, and see themselves as a part of the whole rather than isolated from the rest of the organization. Anxiety diminishes, attention shifts to "we not me," and feelings go from surviving to thriving.

CALMING THE TEMPEST IN THE TEAPOT: MINIMIZING STAFF FEAR AND ANXIETY

Nurse managers have an important role to play in creating safe havens for weathering the storms and the aftermath of organizational change. The following actions go a long way in helping nursing staff manage both large and small-scale change.

1. **Communicate, communicate, and communicate.** Use at least two to three different media to communicate information about change in the workplace. Knowing that staff members differ in their preferences for modes of communication, you may then avoid the ever-favorite response, "Nobody ever tells us anything." Some staff members like written memos while others prefer face-to-face communication. The challenge of effective communication provides an opportunity to become creative. For example, if staff members are younger than 30, why not try text messaging them? But, be careful with e-mails when emotional content is part of or implied in the message. It often fails to convey the tone and nuances of the message.
2. **Establish a mechanism for regular communication updates to keep staff informed.** The more staff members feel they are a part of the information loop, the less powerless they will feel and more likely they will be to continue to support change initiatives, feel respected, and trust in you as their manager.
3. **Create opportunities for staff members to provide feedback on what they heard.** Ask staff what they like about what they heard and what they are not clear about. Ask for their comments or suggestions.
4. **Reinforce reality.** Help staff to understand that proposed changes will happen with or without their permission. That being said, there may be opportunities for staff input for how changes are implemented. It is helpful for staff to know what is negotiable and what is not.
5. **Manage "I heard it through the grapevine!"** Ensure that communication is accurate and timely. Information that travels through the organizational grapevine travels at the speed of light and if false can create unnecessary pain and anxiety. Many rely on grapevine communication without regard for accuracy. Nurse managers can help guide staff to seek out reputable

sources and encourage clarification of misleading information. When someone states "I heard that . . . ," invite that person to check the information for accuracy or offer to do so for them.

6. **Never say "I can't talk about that right now"** when responding to a question from a staff member. Nothing ignites suspicion and generates anxiety faster than a dismissive statement. Staff immediately begin to speculate about why you cannot say anything and, in no time at all, fill the information void with their own interpretation. If you do not know the answer to a question, simply say, "I don't have an answer for you at this time, but I promise as soon as I find out anything I will let you know." Or try, "I don't have the information you are looking for, but I will find out and get back to you by. . . . " If at the end of the specified period you still do not have the information, tell them that and assure them that you are still trying.
7. **Staff can handle the whole truth better than half-truths.** Openness and transparency communicate respect and build trust no matter what the news.

FAST FACTS in a NUTSHELL

- You can never communicate too much during times of change.
- Communication rule: Get the right message to the right person at the right time.

THAT "SOFT, FUZZY STUFF" MATTERS

Managing anxiety, fear, and uncertainty among staff is first a matter of understanding your own reactions to change, naming what you are feeling, and dealing with those feelings, and then tuning into what your staff may be feeling. The steps that nurse managers can take to help staff members manage their anxieties and fears should be premised on trust, mutual respect, and principles of open and transparent communication delivered in an environment of compassion and empathy.

Summary

- Ignoring the feelings of staff may slow the progress of change.
- Managing feelings in response to change builds trust between the manager and staff and hastens staff's engagement in the change process.

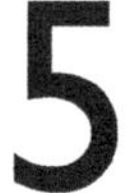

Got Gap?

Managing the Intergenerational Workplace

The complexities of today's changing world of work become more interesting with the presence of at least four generations in the workplace. Managing a mixture of values, life experiences, cultural diversity, and work ethics can either be a nightmare or a dream for nurse managers. When nurse managers are guided by the principle of—and require—respect for all, they lay the foundation for healthy workplace relationships regardless of the generational mix.

In this chapter, you will learn:

1. The key characteristics of the four main cohorts of generations in the workplace: seniors, boomers, Generation Xers, and Generation Ys
2. What each generation values, needs, and is motivated by
3. Strategies for managing multiple generations

THE CHALLENGES OF MANAGING GENERATIONAL COHORTS

With differing life experiences, values, and expectations about work characterizing staff members, the potential for

intergenerational conflict in many of today's workplaces is very real. Staff members can get caught up in sniping at one another with comments such as, "These young nurses don't know anything!" or "Why don't those old ducks just retire and make room for me!" The biggest sources of contention among the different generations lie in their perceptions about levels of educational preparation, work ethic, use of technology, and prior practices and procedures ("the way things used to be done around here"). While generation bashing happens within each cohort, the boomers need to think twice before they bash the Gen Xers and Ys. Why? Because the boomers produced them! Nurse managers who facilitate intergenerational understanding help decrease interpersonal tension, improve the quality of workplace relationships, and promote a spirit of collaboration.

FAST FACTS in a NUTSHELL

- Time spent on generation bashing depletes staff energy, redirects staff focus away from patient care, and flies in the face of the standards of practice, which require nurses to support one another in practice.

KNOW YOUR GENERATIONAL MIX

Nurse managers should have at least a basic understanding of what makes each generation tick and clearly articulated expectations about how all staff members treat one another. With the plethora of available research on the intergenerational workplace, it is easy to become overwhelmed with information about how to manage the members of each cohort. Stuart and Laraia, in their book *Principles and Practice of Psychiatric Nursing* (2000), offer basic principles that capture the fundamentals of relationships with other human beings. By extension these principles (also implicit in codes of ethics) can shape how we behave at work in relation to one another, regardless of the generation we represent. These beliefs provide a useful framework to guide nurse manager's actions in promoting healthy intergenerational relationships.

For Your Consideration: Excellent Principles to Live By

Try using and referring to these principles, adapted from American Psychiatric Nursing Association, to guide relationships among all staff, as well as your relationship with staff:

1. The need for respect is universal among human beings.
2. All individuals have intrinsic worth and dignity.
3. Every individual has the potential to change.
4. All behavior is purposeful and meaningful.

Exploring each of the principles with staff can help establish a framework for how the generations work together. Facilitating staff discussions about how each of these statements would be expressed in their peer group relationships would be inspiring, to say the least.

FAST FACTS in a NUTSHELL

- Regardless of the generation all individuals have a basic need to be treated with dignity and respect.
- Nurse managers must lead and facilitate this process among staff.

INTERESTING TIDBITS ABOUT THE GENERATIONS

The span of years attributed to each generation in the descriptions that follow are not carved in stone. Some individuals possess characteristics from two generational cohorts. The descriptions are, by necessity, brief and intended to whet your appetite for further learning:

Traditionalists, a.k.a. Seniors, Veterans, the Silent Generation (Born Before 1945)

- *Events of influence:* The world wars; the Great Depression.
- *Characteristics:* Hard work, loyalty, sacrifice, thriftiness; working fast to meet deadlines. Expected the workplace to take care of them for life.
- *What nurse managers need to know about them:* They prefer to have decisions explained, and clearly defined structures. They have a tendency for black-and-white thinking, follow procedures exactly as outlined, and require support and recognition of accomplishments.

Baby Boomers (Born Between 1945 and 1965)

- *Events of influence:* Vietnam War, Cold War, assassination of JFK, space exploration, the sexual revolution, drugs, and rock 'n' roll.
- *Characteristics:* Personal fulfillment, optimism, crusades; buy now, pay later; live to work. Since changing jobs frequently was looked upon negatively as a sign of "personal instability," many spent entire careers with the same organization.
- *What nurse managers need to know about them:* Most prefer defined structures, clear expectations, flexibility, and recognition. They want to be left alone! They are disillusioned, tired, and have low to no trust in the workplace. They want their pay and are on a countdown to their pensions. Some are retired and still on the job! Economic realities have forced many adult children of boomers to return to live with their parents, often with *their* families in tow (leading to the coined term "boomerangs"). This recent family phenomenon can create additional financial burdens for seniors and boomers, shooting a hole through Freedom 55 plans and pushing retirement plans into the future.

Generation X (Born Between 1965 and 1980)

- *Events of influence:* These were the first latchkey kids, who often came home to empty houses. Many are from single-parent or dual working-parent families. The energy crisis and turbulent economic times created instability in the job market, leaving this generation to witness the effects of their parents being laid off as companies downsized. In turn, this generation was left with a strong ethic of self-reliance, disillusionment, and little confidence in the belief (unlike their baby boomer parents) that the organization for which they worked would take care of them. (When such organizations have subsequently been criticized by boomers as being disloyal, is it any wonder?)

- *Characteristics:* Well educated, technologically savvy, and independent problem solvers. (They had to be, what with getting lunches on their own, using microwave ovens, and often looking after younger siblings until a parent arrived home.)
- *What nurse managers need to know about them:* They are goal oriented, money focussed, work to live, prefer to work independently, and love project work. They want frequent feedback to determine if their career goals are on track and will change jobs to meet their goals or if they are not treated well. The want rewards (preferably monetary), recognition, flexibility, and a harmonious relationship between work and their personal life.

Generation Y, a.k.a. Millennials (Born After 1980)

- *Events of influence:* Boomers gave them everything, including the latest technology, designer clothes, video games, and tons of praise. They participated in numerous activities as children, were encouraged to express their feelings, and spoke out. Their awareness of global events boggles the mind thanks to their accessibility to instant, 24-hour worldwide news and social media coverage.
- *Characteristics:* They are collaborators, techno wizards, team players, and high performers if motivated, especially if they like you! They have a can-do attitude. They tend not to respond to command-and-control leadership and become easily bored. They want flexibility and respect for their life outside of work, and respond well to change.
- *What nurse managers need to know about them:* They thrive on challenges and can handle more than one task at a time. They expect a coach, a mentor, a friend—not a boss. They want respect, honesty, and to work for ethical and environmentally responsible organizations. And, by the way, they "just wanna have fun."

WHAT THE GENERATIONS CAN OFFER EACH OTHER

1. **Traditionalists/Silent/Veterans:** This generation has seen it all. Because many of them valued loyalty and remained with the organization for decades, they bring the perspective of history to the practice setting. While some younger nurses may regard them as "dinosaurs" in the system, they can also be viewed as sources of inspiration because of their character and experience!
2. **Baby Boomers:** While many Boomers freely admit they are ready to retire, others, especially those now entering their fifties and early sixties, are not, for a number of reasons including meeting financial demands, enjoying their current role, and organizational pressure to remain on the job due to staffing shortages. This generation has been downsized, reengineered, and pummelled with organizational change. Nurse managers must think about the impact of workload and the physical demand being placed on aging baby boomers who choose to extend their work lives. Boomers possess a wealth of knowledge and skills that make them ideal for providing lighter, less demanding, care while serving as mentors and coaches to younger or less experienced staff.
3. **Generation X:** Because they are independent, project oriented, and innovative, members of this generation are natural leaders in implementing or facilitating change in the workplace. While many nurse managers are swamped with numerous commitments, Gen Xers are chomping at the bit, waiting to be asked to assume a project, take charge of a situation, or become your next "Mini-Me" as nurse manager!
4. **Generation Y/Millennials:** These are your "go-to techno wizards," bursting with creativity, wanting to help others, to belong, and to make a difference. Who better to help in the implementation of technology-related to patient care?

JUST TELL ME WHAT YOU WANT—WHAT YOU REALLY, REALLY WANT

Most people regardless of their generation want:

- To be treated with dignity and respect
- To be recognized for jobs well done and told thank you
- To have their needs recognized and understood by their nurse manager

- To receive constructive feedback
- To participate in meaningful work
- To contribute to the greater good
- To be paid fairly

GOT GAP?

Strategies for nurse managers in bridging the generational gap:

- Scan your workplace for the types and numbers in your generational mix.
- Develop a plan to meet the generational communication needs of your staff by reflecting on the tools you currently use for communicating. Are they effective? Is there room for improvement? Ask each staff member for his or her input and ideas.
- Determine how each staff member can best use his or her generation-based strengths to contribute to addressing the challenges in the workplace and improving patient care.
- Be mindful of the underbelly of negative interpersonal dynamics among the generations in your workplace. Especially watch for eyeball rolling!
- Create opportunities for conversations about the generations (e.g., staff meetings or nursing in-services). Discuss how generational differences positively and negatively affect relationships between nurses and patients and among nursing staff.
- If you want to pair the generations on a project or in providing nursing care, try combining a senior and Gen Xer or match a Gen Y with a boomer. These pairings have more in common than you or they may think.
- Manage generation bashing when you hear it by stating something like this, "This is not how we talk about our professional colleagues in our workplace."

FAST FACTS in a NUTSHELL

- How well intergenerational staff members work together will depend on how well the nurse manager engages staff in creating a respectful workplace, understands what makes each generational cohort tick, and inspires staff to believe that together they are better!

CRISIS OR OPPORTUNITY?

The reality for many nurse managers is that intergenerational differences at work can lead to relationship crises or incredible opportunities among staff. It all depends on how they are handled. As a crisis, the situation will invite differing expectations, tension, conflict, hurtful behaviors, and poor quality of care. However, the same situation led and managed by an inspired nurse manager can create opportunities for generational cross-pollination, coaching and mentoring between the generations, creative initiatives for quality improvement, and fun.

Creating opportunities for intergenerational groups to sit down and talk with each other is a healthy way to promote understanding—about what they like about each generation, what behaviors of each generation challenge them, and what strengths each generation brings to the workplace. It also promotes staff learning and professional growth.

. . . and they lived happily ever after.

THE END

FAST FACTS in a NUTSHELL

Summary

- When nurse managers require mutual respect, understanding, and acceptance of diversity among their intergenerational staff, they demonstrate and live the expectations embedded in their codes of ethics and standards of professional practice.

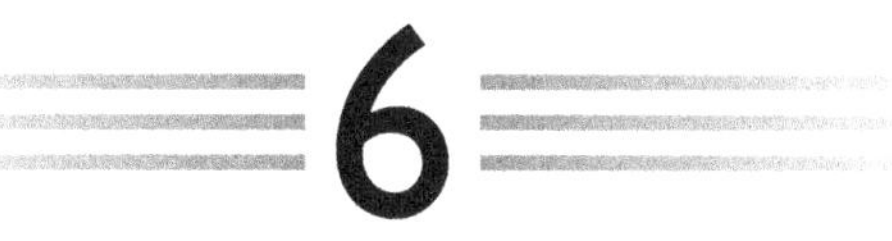

"It Was the Best of Times, It Was the Worst of Times . . ."

Managing and Facilitating Change and Transitions

The ability to facilitate change and manage transitions remains a relatively new competency for nurse managers. Although this area was formerly left to senior leaders and change management gurus, nurse managers had to deal with the fallout from staff transitions. Nurse managers who understand the potential impact of organizational change on the psychological transitions of staff and the workplace culture are better able to respond in a proactive and supportive manner.

In this chapter, you will learn:

1. The importance of understanding the human impact of organizational change
2. How psychological transitions influence staff behaviors in the workplace
3. Strategies for facilitating change in your practice setting

THE METAPHORICAL TRAIN OF CHANGE IS COMIN' DOWN THE TRACK

To truly understand staff's perception of organizational change, view it within the context of the metaphor of the "train is leaving the station." Here, staff are invited to "hop on," baggage and all; lay down on the tracks; or remain on the platform, which by the way is about to be burned! If you can visualize the feelings that accompany this journey such as fear of the unknown and what work will look like at the end of the journey, then you are well on your way to developing a plan for managing change and transition.

THE RIPPLE EFFECT OF ORGANIZATIONAL CHANGE

The degree of impact of organizational change on staff depends on several factors, including the frequency of change, staff experience with past change, and how well change was managed. When change occurs in one part of the organization, other unaffected staff may respond with the casual interest of a bystander. If, however, the change is imposed on them, staff members may respond in a variety of ways, including feelings ranging from joy and indifference to powerlessness, grief, and anger. Sometimes the presence of these feelings is not obvious. When negative feelings surface the quality of work life takes a direct hit as the atmosphere is dominated by anger, frustration, apathy, low self-esteem, resistance to change, and infighting.

At the same time, the work ethic of caring that staff normally extend to their peers, patients, and clients may assume a narrower focus if their energies are directed exclusively toward patient care and self-preservation. This situation leaves staff with little room or interest in supporting their colleagues and organizational change imperatives.

NURSES' ANGER

Nurse managers must recognize the depth of emotions staff members have about work and female nurses' potential for harboring deep-seated, often unexpressed anger. Research on women's anger has not been extensive. Thomas, Smucker, and Droppleman (1998) shed light on the fact that **anger develops in women as**

the result of an accumulation of feelings associated with "hurt, frustration and disillusionment" (p. 311). They also describe the medical impact of nurses' unresolved anger, which may lead to conditions such as hypertension, obesity, and migraine headaches. **For nurse managers it may be of more than a passing interest to note the possibility of a connection between organizational change, nurses' anger, the health of nurses, and quality of work life.**

KNOW YOUR WORKPLACE CULTURE

As nurse manager, how do you help nurses step back from the demands of a changing, hectic workplace and acknowledge their situation, name their feelings, and restore their sense of caring power when organizational pressures are bearing down?

One strategy is **to conduct a cultural assessment of your practice setting** to determine staff readiness to accept change. Once you determine where staff fit on the acceptance scale, you can identify what staff will need to engage in the change process. The following questions may help you identify potential "hot spots" and point you toward some steps to help staff adapt to and embrace a new way of being:

- How content are staff members? In other words, what is their degree of nattering?
- How well do staff work together?
- Is there a spirit of cooperation, collaboration, and support or is there conflict, tension, and in-fighting?
- If you sense or observe resistance, what is its source? Are staff members fed up, tired, burned out, lacking trust in the process?
- Who may be resisting and why?
- Who are the formal and informal leaders among your staff? Who is working with you and who is not?
- What kind of influence do these leaders exert?
- Which staff members are most likely to support organizational change? Who are your champions of change?
- What roles can these change-ready staff members play in positively influencing others?

- What type of language is reflected in your workplace? Is it upbeat, positive, and professional, or does it reflect, negativity, victimization, and resistance? Are there frequent references to "them" or "they"? Do staff members complain to patients and clients?

SMART MESSENGERS DON'T GET SHOT

Tis a perilous journey one takes when delivering a message of impending change. But it does not have to be so. The following scenario may help you in crafting and delivering a message of change:

> Your practice area is about to be affected by a dramatic organizational change process. As part of this change, the service will now include treatment of patients who were formerly treated in another location. There will be no reductions in staffing.

How would you communicate and prepare staff members for acceptance and engagement and lay the groundwork for change with the least amount of disruption and upheaval? How could you make this change happen as smoothly as possible with the least amount of disruption and upheaval? The following ponderables are for your consideration.

DON'T TELL: FACILITATE!

As you think about managing change that affects your practice setting, be aware that **a more traditional command-and-control style of leading is less effective than facilitating, coaching, mentoring, and yes, counseling.** Recall the Chinese proverb, "Tell me and I may forget; show me and I may remember; involve me and I will understand."

When organizational change is imposed, nurse managers may have little time to learn expert skills to facilitate the process. They can, however, draw upon principles of therapeutic communication in helping staff manage a new workplace reality. According to Freire (1997), facilitation creates an environment in which individuals are helped to name their experiences, engage in dialogue about their situation, and transform their world. How do you find the time to create these opportunities? The real question that requires an answer is not how, but when?

- Facilitating true dialogue creates opportunities for reflection, empathic listening, exchanging ideas, laughter, and professional growth.
- Dialogue opens the door for increased self-awareness and promotes camaraderie.

CRASH COURSE IN FACILITATION 101

Nurses are natural facilitators. Here is a refresher on how you do it—your crash course in facilitation. **Facilitation is a process that requires you to help participants assess their needs, encourage meaningful conversations, develop collaborative interventions, strengthen workplace relationships, and create positive outcomes that benefit all.**

1. Consider the following metaphor and visualize your entire staff sitting before you as a patient who is facing surgery and expressing fear, denial, and anger. What nursing diagnoses would you attribute to "your patient"? What would your nursing interventions include? What outcomes would you anticipate? How would you evaluate the outcomes?
2. Develop your plan for facilitation, create opportunities for dialogue (roundtable discussions work great), invite feedback from small groups to share with the larger group, listen for key messages, listen for what is not being said, help staff distill their messages, and facilitate the development on an action plan and steps for follow-up. Basically listen more than you speak; repeat what they said for clarification ("This is what I hear you saying . . . Is that correct?"), and write down what they say.
3. For change to be accepted staff will need:
   - A compelling reason to change. Help staff answer the question, "Why change?"
   - Lots of information to support the reason for change, such as data and stories.
   - Opportunities to become involved.
   - Communication, communication, and more communication.
   - More than memos. Staff could be drowning in them and someone will say, with just a hint of indignation, "I never saw that!"

- Clear expectations. Tell them what you expect from them and from yourself. Ask for their feedback to determine if your expectations of your role are consistent with theirs.
- Opportunities to celebrate small and big successes.
- Empathy for their thoughts and feelings.
- Positive role modeling on your part may be the most powerful way to ensure staff remain on the path forward. Share some of your experiences and keep the focus positive.
- Knowledge that, bottom line, this is the direction the organization is heading in and as employees they are responsible for engaging in the process. If they cannot or will not, then it is time to consider employment alternatives.

This is not intended to be an all-inclusive list, but it will give you an idea of what to look for and include in your own and staff's journey toward successful implementation. Once you have assessed the workplace culture and staff's state of readiness for change, you can develop a collaborative plan of action that supports change initiatives.

SNAGS, ROADBLOCKS, AND WORKPLACE VARMINTS

We all know the expression, "The best laid plans of mice and men. . . . " Therefore, **expect the best of outcomes in planned change but do not be surprised if an obstacle rears its ugly head**. Delays happen as well. When these occur, remind yourself that you have a choice in how you view the situation. It can be either a crisis or an opportunity! Sometimes snags are blessings in disguise. Instead of getting your knickers in a twist, step back and ask yourself, "What are the opportunities and possibilities that exist right now at this moment?" Think about it, and then seize the moment!

Remember, during the implementation of your plan: be creative, listen well, and be empathetic. However, also remember that it is your job to inspire and support staff in achieving the goal. Face-to-face meetings are the best venue for communicating with staff. Offer bulleted lists that include "just the facts, Ma'am" and any other strategies that you can conjure up to grab the attention of your intergenerational staff members and hold their interest. One more thing: If your sense of humor is dormant, wake it up!

FOLLOW THE LEADER: LEADING CHANGE

If you are tasked with the responsibility for leading a change initiative, know that your greatest challenge will come not from the hard issues related to the design or developmental phases of change management but from the soft or human response. In the end, **successful change management is less about processes and operations and more about managing the mindsets of staff** to prepare and fully engage them in quality improvement processes.

Several excellent templates are available to guide you in planning the formal change management process. John Kotter, Peter Block, William Bridges, and Rick Maurer all offer excellent models and valuable insights into managing change, steps to be taken, guides for conversations, achieving engagement, and managing resistance.

CHANGE CAN BE HARD; TRANSITIONS CAN BE HARDER

One of the toughest realities for managers and staff to accept is the constancy of change. Just as orange is the new black, change is the new normal. When change and the ensuing psychological transitions are managed well, nurse managers and their staffs achieve both a strategic and patient care advantage. When you are prepared to expect and manage a variety of reactions from staff do not neglect your own transitions.

MANAGING CHANGE IS ABOUT MANAGING MINDSETS

- In a changing workplace, we are all on a learning curve toward a paradigm shift that will transform how we think about work and how we get the work done.
- We have the power to choose our attitude.
- Attitude is a symptom of a psychological mindset.
- Mindsets include our self-concept, values, self-esteem, beliefs, as well as how we perceive our world.
- Deal with your mindset first and then with that of your staff.

KNOWLEDGE IS POWER

The more we know about the change process and the psychological transitions we go through in response to change, the more prepared we are to prevent and manage unhealthy staff responses, poor quality of care, and deteriorating quality of work life. As human beings, we are inclined to be creatures of habit. Thus, when change is anticipated or introduced we react with a broad range of thoughts, feelings, and behaviors ranging from joy to despair. William Bridges was among the first to identify the human response to organizational change. His seminal book, *Managing Transitions: Making the Most of Change* (1991), was written in the early 1990s when there were few books on the subject. Although many excellent reference books have since been written on change management, Bridges offers user-friendly ponderables for your consideration and a practical framework for helping managers and staff navigate the change process, weather the storms of transitions, see the possibilities, celebrate successes, and prepare for the next round of change.

FAST FACTS in a NUTSHELL

- According to William Bridges (1991), Humans + Change = Psychological Transition.
- Transition is a psychological process that individuals go through to manage and adapt to change.

WHEN CHANGE BEGINS, TRANSITIONS FOLLOW

Change is inevitable in today's workplaces, but **change without successful transition initiatives can be doomed to failure.** According to Bridges, every change is accompanied by a psychological response, the transition process, which consists of Endings, Neutral Zone, and New Beginnings. The rate at which individuals progress through the three phases of the process will vary among staff. Transition occurs whether change is perceived as a good or bad change. While some staff will hold onto the past by refusing to move forward, others will progress along the transition continuum toward the next phase, where chaos and confusion are the order of the day as staff members struggle to accommodate the changes they are required to make. Eventually, most staff will embrace their new way of being and working.

The next three chapters create opportunities to enlighten nurse managers about key behaviors typically observed on the transition continuum and how to manage them.

FAST FACTS in a NUTSHELL

Summary

- The more nurse managers know about facilitating and managing the change process, the more likely staff members are to engage successfully in the change initiative.
- Regard change management as a road trip to your practice setting's future. Some roads will be like the autobahn; some will be rocky and less traveled; some will beg for further exploration; others will downright scare you, causing you to turn back and correct course. No matter which road you travel, the experiences will enrich your management learning journey.

REFERENCES

Bridges, W. (1991). *Managing transitions: Making the most of change.* Reading, MA: Perseus Books.

Freire, P. (1997). *Pedagogy of the oppressed.* New York, NY: Continuum.

Thomas, S., Smucker, C., & Droppleman, P. (1998). It hurts most around the heart: A phenomenological exploration of women's anger. *Journal of Advanced Nursing, 28*(2), 311–322.

It's Over

Managing the End of Old Ways of Being

One of the advantages of good teamwork is the familiarity that team members have with one another. They know whom to call upon when they need help, a good laugh, a shoulder to cry on, or to celebrate their successes. When change is introduced, routines and staff relationships are often disrupted or severed. This chapter outlines common staff responses and offers explanations and strategies for helping staff manage what happens when the once familiar is gone.

In this chapter, you will learn:

1. What happens when the former way of being must give way to the new
2. What behaviors to look for when staff is face with the end of what once was familiar
3. Tips for helping staff let go of the past

THE TRAIN HAS LEFT THE STATION: ONE JOURNEY ENDS, ANOTHER BEGINS

The old way of being is no more! It is over. Depending on the significance of the impending change, these words can create

no response, a mere ripple, or send shock waves through an organization or workplace. Even though this may be anticipated when changes affect clinical practice or workplace relationships, staff will still react. Some will be excited about the possibilities that change can bring, while others may experience disbelief, betrayal, anger, grief, loss, fear, or a combination of these responses.

BIG MISTAKE

With the announcement of impending organizational change, well-meaning leaders invest a great deal of energy carefully crafting the message in such a way as to get staff "buy-in." They may attempt to rally the troops with the familiar battle cry, "People, the train is leaving the station." When staff members hear this, they will probably feel railroaded into accepting the impending change, and feelings of suspicion, anger, resistance, and powerlessness will take hold. Resistance is guaranteed.

IT'S NOT WHAT YOU HEAR, IT'S WHAT YOU DON'T HEAR THAT COUNTS

As you consider communication about change, keep in mind that verbal communication comprises only 7% of an interpersonal interaction. Therefore, **staff members' verbal responses of support to messages about change may mask underlying and unexpressed feelings.** During this time, nurse managers are well advised to listen carefully to what staff is not saying, observe nonverbal actions, and be open to many fascinating reactions.

FASCINATING COMMENTS YOU MAY HEAR

1. "But It Ain't Broke, Why Fix It?"

When staff is overheard making the remark, "it ain't broke," it is a clear signal of a communication gap between the intent of the message and what is perceived. It may also reflect blame that staff members are inclined to assign when they do not see the benefit of impending change. Some nurse managers will mistakenly try to convince staff that their perceptions are wrong when they hear these comments. Sadly, all this accomplishes is to drive the comments underground, shut down communication between the manager and staff, or fuel the fires of "our manager doesn't understand."

2. "Another Flavor of the Month"

Depending on the amount and frequency of change staff has experienced, they may react with a high degree of cynicism. Do not be surprised. They may refer to the pronouncement as a "flavor-of-the-month" initiative. This usually indicates that staff does not see the value of the proposed change and has little faith in a successful outcome. This remark also speaks to a lack of trust in leadership. What staff may really be saying is, "I do not see the need for this change" or "I don't have enough information" or "I don't understand" or "I don't trust you"—or a combination of all of these responses!

3. "I Can't Believe This! Where Is This Coming From?"

This response can reflect staff's level of awareness about what is happening in the broader organization, the timing of the message, or how the message is delivered.

4. "Been There, Done That, Bought the T-Shirt."

While a comment like this seems resistant and dismissive, it actually serves as a cue that the information received may not be what was intended or that this most recent change is no change at all in the minds of some. Some staff members have been around long enough to believe that they have "seen and done it all." The danger lies in their potential to influence others in a negative way.

How much this remark influences the peer group depends on how much power the individual has.

THINGS YOU MAY SEE

Breaking Up Is Hard to Do

Many staff will state that their peer group at work is like their second family. When staff groups are forced to separate due to restructuring, the loss can be so profound that the grief and anger can last for years. Anger toward management's decision to make these changes can be intense.

Some staff members have more to lose than others when the group membership is altered or disbanded. Depending on the nature of their workplace relationships, some individuals will lose real or perceived power and status. This can be threatening not only to the individual who has the power but also to group members, who may believe they have lost their informal leader. Losing more than one staff member can create a powerful grief reaction among remaining staff. When the sense of loss at work is this severe the potential for individual and group depression is very real. Change cannot successfully be absorbed until the underlying issues related to grief and loss are dealt with in a compassionate manner.

When the Nurse Manager Is Downsized or Redeployed

Grief among staff members is experienced during real or perceived loss, and the effects can be vast. Left unmanaged, its toll becomes apparent in staff relationships. Chronically negative workplace relationships emanating from unresolved grief can result in a mindset that a replacement manager will never fill the void. Successive nurse managers may face huge resistance and staff rejection than can persist for years. Dealing with this type of anger and loss will require patience, understanding, skilful handling, and refocusing of staff members' attention on their patients and professional practice.

Fear of the Unknown

Many staffs have a high need for order and predictability. Not knowing what lies ahead can induce mild to severe anxiety and behaviors that reflect any number of symptoms, including decreased productivity, complaining, irritability, and increasing use of sick time. Fear of making a career-limiting move may cause some staff to become non-participative, go through the motions, or mentally "shut down."

Real and Perceived Loss

It is safe to assume that there may be numerous real and perceived losses experienced when traditional ways of performing a task or procedure change, familiar staff are relocated, or a department is closed and a new location is opened. Loss can be associated with the threat of or actual job loss, personal or professional status (because of role or job change), peer group power dynamics, giving up the familiar, and the introduction of new equipment, processes, or care delivery.

When Staff "Families" Blend

This process is a huge adjustment for all concerned, cannot be fixed quickly, and the process for integration closely rivals that of the challenges of blending families after divorce. Patience, compassion, and humor are key.

FAST FACTS in a NUTSHELL

- When a way of being is over, staff may struggle with losing or changing familiar patterns, issues of power and control, relationships, and ways of thinking and acting.
- Whatever staff members perceive is their reality. The language staff uses to express these perceptions should never be dismissed lightly. It is the nurse manager's job to help staff express and name what lies beneath their seemingly offhand remarks.

THREE STATEMENTS YOU SHOULD NEVER UTTER WHEN SOMETHING ENDS

Guaranteed, you will shake staff's sense of trust in you if you say any of the following things:

1. **You**: "Trust me; this change will be a good thing."
   Staff's unspoken response: "No we won't trust you. You are management's messenger. You report to senior management, and they have the power to fire you and us."
2. **You**: "We need your buy-in."
   Staff's unspoken response: "I am not so sure I want to buy anything right now. You sound like a shady used car salesman, and who trusts them?"
3. **You**: "I can't talk about this right now."
   Staff's unspoken response: "Hmmm. There must be something they're holding back. They are probably going to fire us all or close our service. I better start looking for another job. You can never really trust management!"
4. **You**: "Don't worry!"
   Staff's unspoken response: "Easy for you to say, you're management!"

TIPS FOR LETTING GO

1. Reflect on your position within the context of endings. Do you support the proposed changes? How do you go through the motions of supporting change when you do not support the strategy? How will that influence staff? What do you need to do to manage your personal acceptance of the proposed changes? What resources do you need to call upon to support you and the staff as you move forward?
2. Tell the truth.
3. Acknowledge and manage your own and staff's anger and grief associated with loss.
4. Help staff to reflect on and let go of the past. What was good about the old way of being? What needed improvement? Explore with staff how the new changes could lead to improvement consistent with their own thinking.
5. Manage overt and covert resistance.

6. Create an open-door policy so that staff members can drop in to express their feelings. When they do, help them to determine what steps are necessary for them to move forward.
7. Reinforce reality by giving staff information, data, costs, and other details. If the change is about the bottom line, show staff your budget printouts.
8. Ask the question, "Why change?" And then ask staff members to answer it.
9. Provide staff with a brief bulleted list of the key points you want communicated and the overall organizational plan (no more than six points on a page) for moving forward.
10. Remind them that accepting change is uncomfortable for most of us. It is okay for us to feel what we do for a while, but all of us have to move on sooner rather than later.
11. Commit to communicate, communicate, and communicate. (Tell; write; tell again.)
12. Make yourself available to answer questions. Discourage the use of the grapevine, and encourage staff members to come to you or check things out themselves.
13. If you do not know the answer to a question, tell them so and that you will find out and get back to them as soon as possible.
14. If change is going to alter your unit culture or staff mix by introducing more staff or moving staff to other areas, gather the staff together before the change occurs and discuss the following:
    - What are the accomplishments we are most proud of as a unit?
    - What improvements do we feel need to happen to improve our practice or service quality?
    - How will the impending changes improve our services?
    - What obstacles might we face during this improvement?
    - What plans can we make to celebrate our past?

15. Remember: It is not what you say; it is what you do. Staff will be watching you very closely to see if your actions match your words. (How upbeat are you about these changes? Do your words and actions reflect support for the organization's direction? If you are frustrated about more change, is it showing?)

Suggestions for celebrating what once was: Create a scrapbook or a photo album of past events, or create a social event to celebrate the past and welcome the future.

Summary

- Successfully managing change from a former way of being is mostly about managing the mindset of staff members. The "soft" issues frequently associated with change are fear, letting go, grief and loss, celebrating and honoring the past, and paving the way to the new normal of chaos and confusion.
- This is the new normal. Staff need your leadership more than ever at this critical time.

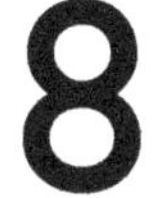

Now What?

Managing Chaos and Confusion

Once change has been introduced to your staff as inevitable, your main task and that of staff is to "make it work." Meet your new best friends: chaos and confusion! This chapter describes some of the antics that staff members may craft in response to their emerging new reality, and tips for managing their innovative and occasionally challenging behavior.

In this chapter, you will learn:

1. How chaos and confusion impacts staff as they move through the second phase of transition toward a new way of being.
2. Tips for managing chaos and confusion.

THE PERILOUS JOURNEY OF CHAOS AND CONFUSION ON THE BIG THUNDER MOUNTAIN RAILROAD

If you have ever taken Disneyland's Big Thunder Mountain railroad ride, you have been initiated into a world of surprises, obstacles, and exhilaration. This experience is not unlike the new world that can follow the introduction of planned change. The metaphorical train of change has left the station loaded with a mix of anxious, excited, and a few reluctant passengers. They are embarking on a journey but are unsure what the destination will look like. Little do they know that along the way they may face perils of frightening proportions. They know that they cannot turn back, and they expect the trip to get worse before it gets better.

Remember the boulders that threatened to crush you on the Disneyland ride? The train's steep, slow climb up the mountain and rapid and shaky descent? Crossing the ravine on the rickety bridge before finally reaching the station? As the passengers jumped off the train, most were smiling and excited. Some disembarked dazed and shaken. In a few instances, a small number of brave passengers quickly ran to catch the next train for another exciting ride! This pretty much sums up the second phase of the journey of transition between endings and new beginnings.

As the metaphorical conductor, your job is to make the passengers are as comfortable as possible in the learning journey ahead; in other words, to support staff as they prepare for things to get messy, uncomfortable, and at times simply wretched! Knowing this phase can be rough gives you a heads-up on how to manage the obstacles you may face. This phase of transition is characterized by chaos, confusion, and potential nastiness, underpinned with a modicum of anticipation.

THINGS YOU MAY HEAR ALONG THE JOURNEY OF CHAOS AND CONFUSION

1. "H-E-L-L-L-P!"

2. "Just Tell Us What to Do!"

In the muck and mire of chaos and confusion, frustration can be the norm. Feelings of powerlessness play out in a number of ways. In particular, the drama associated with merging staff is played out through territorial battles, power struggles, and competition. In-fighting can distract from the work.

3. "Show Me the Policy!"

When departments or organizations merge, multiple policy and procedure manuals are supposed to merge as well, but this rarely happens fast enough. In the meantime when nurses are challenged by a practice issue and go looking for the correct policy or procedure to follow, they may find several or none. When this happens, staff can feel confused, anxious, frustrated, and fearful for patient safety.

4. "That's Not My Job. If You Make Me Do It, I'll Grieve!"

This "line in the sand" response is an indicator of the level of distress staff members feel as they move through this tumultuous period. They are looking for anything to hold onto, to reassure them that they are okay and their patients are safe. Despite solid plans and implementation strategies being in place, there are no sure-fire rules for managing successful change. A book by Warren Bennis, *Managing People Is Like Herding Cats!* (1999) captures the essence of managing people during organizational change. At this time, there are only guidelines.

5. "I'm Tired of All This Change. I Just Want to Nurse My Patients!"

Staff members are more inclined to withdraw into themselves during this phase. They become "me" focused and have little energy to spread around. They are in survival mode, and their morale may plummet. They may feel patients are being cheated of quality care and feel guilty about it, but not necessarily motivated enough to change.

6. "I Don't Like This. I Want to Go Back to the Good ol' Days."

Wanting to return to the familiar is natural. What is not natural is to sabotage progress or to be angry enough to negate change efforts.

THINGS YOU MAY SEE

Polarized Staff

If change requires you to bring two or more distinct staff groups together, expect that their natural inclination will be to band together in their groups of origin. Turf wars, competition about who is the better group of nurses, and nasty comments are all expressions of staff's struggles with adapting to a new way of being. Teamwork temporarily goes the way of the dodo bird. (Unlike the bird, it will return!)

Increased Use of Sick Time

Mixed emotions, accommodating different practices, and mental and physical exhaustion can cause staff to more readily call in sick and feel less inclined to go the proverbial extra mile.

Following the Informal Leader

According to Bridges, this is when people struggle with ambiguity, look for answers that not be there, and readily attach themselves to someone who is authoritative, seems to know what they are doing, and appears competent and confident (1991, p. 39). This is fine, as long as this newfound and informal leader is positive, proactive, and aligned with the direction of the organization. If this person is negative, reactive, and challenging your leadership, you may be facing a potential power struggle of mythic proportions. Bring it on!

FAST FACTS in a NUTSHELL

- Staff members are more willing to embrace change when they see how it will improve practice, patient care, or processes.
- There are always a few staff members who can only focus on themselves. They try to maintain the status quo and just wait it out, longing for things to "return to normal."

THE GOOD NEWS

When staff members recognize that tension among them is energy zapping and decide to work together for the good of patients, the seeds are sown for collaboration, cooperation, and creativity in the newly defined workplace. Focusing on their collective strengths and moving past what is wrong is a clear sign of a shift in mindset. The train is headed for solid ground.

FAST FACTS in a NUTSHELL

- Expect chaos and confusion in between what was and what will be.
- During the phase of chaos and confusion, staff members may look for answers when there are none.
- Things will get better.

MANAGING CHAOS AND CONFUSION, AND ANYTHING ELSE THROWN YOUR WAY

1. Reinforce reality by clearly communicating the following messages to staff members:
   - Yes, this is difficult but we have to move forward.
   - Determine whether *you* are thriving or merely surviving.
   - Ask staff if they are merely surviving the journey or are thriving.
   - Ask them what surviving looks like, and then ask them what thriving looks like.
   - Recommend that they choose to thrive!
   - Talk about actions and behaviors that support thriving.
   - Tell staff members that they have the power to choose their attitude on this journey.
   - Remind staff that when organizational change occurs, some decisions are negotiable, and some are not. Individuals may have input into how something is done, but they may not have the authority to determine whether something will be done. Make sure staff understands which is which!

2. Educate staff about transitions.
3. Set both short-term and long-term goals for implementation of initiatives.
4. Look for opportunities to identify emerging leaders and provide opportunities for leadership experiences.
5. Clarify what policies and procedures must be followed at this time. Explain that they are never a substitute for critical thinking and professional practice.
6. Check your generation mix: Have you got a Gen Xer leading an initiative or with a project team? Did you pair your Gen Ys with some boomers?
7. Continue regular verbal and written feedback and acknowledge successes.
8. Be available and visible to help individuals maintain their focus on patient care while implementing change.
9. When staff members seem stuck or the "go forward" plan gets derailed, offer a time-out to review why things are off track and invite their input with an invitation: "Let's figure out how we can get back on track."
10. In collaboration with staff create activities and celebrations that promote connections and collegiality.
11. Have a conversation with staff about the challenges of working to full scope and meeting standards of practice at this time, and how staff is meeting those challenges. Determine if there is a role for you at the unit or organizational level in removing practice barriers.
12. Reinforce that there are no mistakes; there are only opportunities to learn as you make your way through this change.
13. Continue with regular meetings for communication updates.
14. Conduct a self check-in about how you are feeling. Reflect on your self-care strategy.

NEWS FLASH! YOU ARE NOT PERFECT, YOU ARE ONLY HUMAN

Sometimes your plate can be too full as you try to be all things to all people. You feel that if anyone asks you to do one more thing, you might just explode. If you fear that this is the case, you may have to pull the emergency brake, take stock of what you have onboard, shift your cargo, or make some priority decisions about what can temporarily be left behind.

Unless you strongly believe that you might be making a career-limiting move, discuss this situation (using a written plan) with the person to whom you report using the following format:

1. Identify the issue of overload and give examples.
2. State why it is important to address this issue.
3. Describe what benefits would result from a "course correct."
4. Identify anticipated outcomes.
5. Identify timelines for completion.
6. Tell your boss you will give regular updates on your progress.
7. Once your plan is approved, share it with staff.

FAST FACTS in a NUTSHELL

- When you take on too much and try to please everyone, you end up paying a high price. The inability to recognize when you are experiencing work overload can lead to the breakdown of change processes, workplace relationships, and quite possibly, you!
- Just say "No," in the nicest possible way. Although it may seem difficult to say, it is, after all, only a one-syllable word!

ARRIVING AT YOUR NEW DESTINATION

As you and the staff get closer to your destination, take pride in your progress, how well you thrived in your journey, and the realization that as a group, you just might be better now than you were before. You will experience more positive behavior among most of the staff as you settle in and become comfortable with your new way of being. There may be a few staff who have not engaged, and they are the focus of future discussion.

The bottom line is that once you have mastered the chaos and confusion and completed the journey, the worst is over until the next set of changes comes knocking at your door.

Summary

- When the train of organizational change traverses the perilous terrain of chaos and confusion, it eventually reaches its destination. When that happens, pat your back, celebrate the journey, and prepare for a new way of being, new collaborative relationships, and improved outcomes in service delivery. What's not to like?

REFERENCES

Bennis, W. (1999). *Managing people is like herding cats.* Provo, UT: Executive Excellence Publishing.

Bridges, W. (1991). *Managing transitions: Making the most of change.* Reading, MA: Perseus Books.

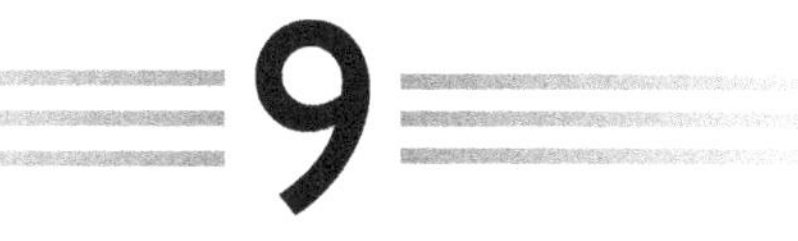

From Isolation to Collaboration

Managing a New Way of Being

Once you have managed the predictable chaos and confusion over the introduction of something or someone new you can expect a period of respite in which calm and serenity prevail. Be assured that it will only last until the next round of change. This chapter celebrates movement away from egocentricity and chaos and toward alignment, collaboration, and overall acceptance of a new way of being.

In this chapter, you will learn:

1. The signs that change is beginning to embed
2. Strategies for managing the beginning of a new way of being

A NEW WAY OF BEING IS JUST OVER THE HORIZON

Managing your own and staff transitions is one of the most difficult challenges facing nurse managers. After this phase is completed, do not be fooled into thinking that the implementation and embedding of the changes is the "easy part." Do not compare it to the challenges you faced in ending the old ways of being and helping individuals work through the confusion that occurs when systems, ideologies, or practices collide. Being tuned into the psychological impact of changes at work provides you and your staff with opportunities for new learning, personal growth, and the chance to make meaningful change.

With chaos and confusion diminishing and territorial battles won and lost, staff members begin to accept the inevitable—that a new way of being is at hand. Whole-scale acceptance by and engagement of all staff is unlikely and will vary among staff in the early stages of the new beginning. When the uptake is slow or becomes temporarily derailed, some cynics may shout with glee, "I told you this wouldn't work!" More likely, they will develop a knowing smile as they pass you in the hallway.

Depending on the mindset of the naysayers and resistors, the implementation and embedding phase may be at risk for complete failure as the potential for a renewed power struggle lurks on the sidelines.

THE PROBLEM WITH IMPLEMENTING PLANNED CHANGE

When planned change takes place there is usually a strategic planning committee hovering in the background, much like a family anticipating the birth of a first child. Ready to assist in the delivery is an appointed steering committee, whose job is to manage and support the process according to meticulously drafted protocols, benchmarks, and tight time lines. The committee's accountability is evidenced in monitoring the course of actions and making course corrections to ensure the "deliverable" arrives on schedule. **However, although the implementation plan and schedule may work in theory, the progression of people along the theoretical continuum is anything but linear and predictable.** Despite "the best laid plans of mice and men," plans can go awry.

- Accepting the inevitable—that plans will run amok, timelines will become moving targets, and people won't do what they are supposed to do for a variety of reasons—better prepares you to manage the beginning of new way of being.
- Managing your own response as you lead your staff during this phase will require you to call upon a number of competencies that include flexibility, patience, resurrecting your sense of humor, maintaining a presence, and living in the moment.

WILL THE PLANNED CHANGE STICK?

That depends. **Do not be surprised if, while the change initiative is still in its infancy, some staff revert to old habits and ways of being.** For example, if you are introducing an automated system, staff may secretly use their tried-and-true handwritten manual system! This behavior may signal any number of things, including resistance, testing the system for permanency, or testing you. In a system where staff members are bombarded by what they perceive as "flavor-of-the-month" changes it makes sense for them to test whether or not this change is "for real." The sooner you identify this behavior, the sooner you can move on.

WHAT YOU MAY EXPERIENCE AS YOU AND YOUR STAFF ENGAGE IN A NEW WAY OF BEING

- The focus of staff energy and caring returns to the patient or client.
- Staff appears more connected to one another.
- Relationships become collaborative rather than territorial.
- The sound of appropriate laughter in your workplace or cafeteria becomes music to your ears.

- Mixed emotions of excitement and anticipatory anxiety emerge during the launch phase and embedding of changes. Note to self: This is normal.
- Staff members who play a part in developing and implementing the "new way of being" develop a greater sense of ownership and pride in the process and outcomes.
- The leadership potential of individual staff members surfaces.
- Staff members who participate on steering committees with others from across the organization begin to expand their workplace horizons by grasping the "big picture" of the interconnectedness of the organization as a whole.
- The potential for staff to become ambassadors of change increases when they see the value of progress as it relates to their practice and quality of care processes.
- Committed and engaged staff become role models for their peers and may inspire others to become involved in future initiatives
- As staff are encouraged and supported in moving though transitions, there is a greater likelihood for personal and professional transformation.

A REFLECTION FOR YOU

"Yesterday is history; tomorrow is a mystery; today is all we have" (unknown source). Throughout the change process, this statement can provide a measure of comfort for both you and the staff as you engage in change and move toward a new way of being. Focusing on the present serves to remind you, staff, and the occasional organizational leader of your individual and collective primary "patients first" responsibility. It is interesting to note that today's organizational literature is placing great emphasis on the importance of presence and mindfulness in clinical practice.

TIPS FOR MANAGING STAFF AS THEY EMBARK AND ENGAGE IN A NEW WAY OF BEING

1. Teach and reinforce the principles of managing change, emphasizing that things may not be perfect yet, everyone is

embarking on a learning curve, and they may have to be willing to take a leap of faith. Ask them to be patient as you tread boldly where few have gone before!

2. Assess staff members' level of engagement in their new way of being by inviting discussion that highlights improvements in care and potential opportunities to identify a topic for nursing research or to produce a scholarly article.
3. Create opportunities for feedback on what is working well, what is not working well, and what could be done better.
4. Review where everyone was in the good ol' days, and "how far we've come." Note achievements and challenges.
5. Initiate a mentoring program.
6. Maintain visibility. Just seeing you in the workplace can quell feelings of uncertainty and anxiety.
7. Create opportunities for ongoing feedback.
8. Continue to talk about and inform staff about the future as you see it— the challenges that you face as manager, the challenges that you all face as a staff, and the challenges that face the organization.
9. Communicate to staff that despite uncertainties, staff members must continue to respect and value one another and work collaboratively. Talk about what working collaboratively looks like. Tell them you will to the best of your abilities be available to support their continuing transitions. (Posting your schedule is helpful.)
10. Help staff to celebrate their success.
11. Remember to say thank you for specific staff achievements and if you can, handwrite thank-you notes.
12. Hop on the leadership bandwagon! When staff demonstrates leadership during the implementation, take note and look for other opportunities for individuals to further develop their newfound skills.
13. Keep your eyes open for lingering resistance or negative attitudes and manage them.
14. Continue to monitor the quality of patient/client care.
15. Tell staff that this is probably not the last they will see and experience organizational change.

Helping staff navigate transitions is one of the most important competencies for nurse managers. Issues related to transitions may be the largest stumbling block to successful change management, professional practice, and healthy workplace relationships.

Yet successfully managing transitions remains an area in which few managers have a great level of comfort and with which many organizations continue to struggle. Equally important for nurse managers is being able to manage their own transitions when they feel they are "caught between a rock and a hard place" as they struggle to balance the demands of staff and those of the organization. Leading change requires nurse managers to be self-aware, flexible, risk takers, innovators, and creative. As such they model the new competencies for a changing world and how to thrive in a changing workplace.

FAST FACTS in a NUTSHELL

Summary

- No one person has all the answers for solving today's complex workplace challenges.
- There is no template for how we proceed toward a new way of being. We've never been here before.
- Since we've never been here before, the only way forward is to work together and do what needs to be done in order to make the necessary changes happen.

PART

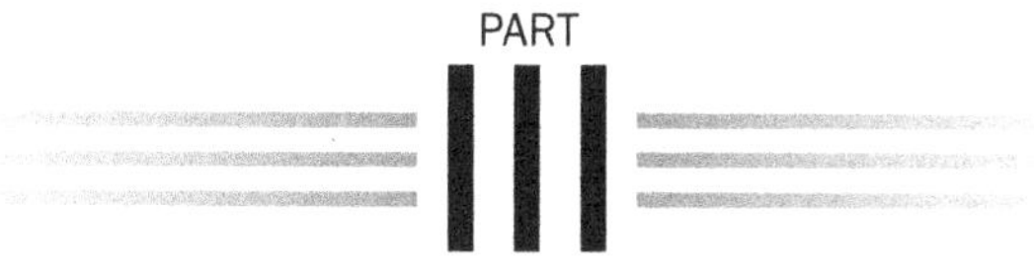

III

Staff Gone Wild?

Managing Your Cast of Characters

10 Got Resistance?

Expect It! Welcome It! Manage It!

Welcome to the murky, energy-sapping world of resistance, with its cast of shady characters. How do you recognize and manage overt and covert forms of resistance? This chapter outlines what to look for and how to handle behaviors that can spell trouble if ignored.

In this chapter, you will learn:

1. Resistance is a normal part of change that creates crises and opportunities
2. The 20/60/20 Rule of Resistance
3. Basic principles and strategies for removing the masks of resistance

RESISTANCE IS A NATURAL PARTNER OF CHANGE

Change is inevitable, and so is resistance to it. People resist for any number of reasons, and nurse managers need to recognize it, understand the reasons, and then manage the behaviors. Unchecked resistance can have a negative impact on the quality of patient care and staff relationships, and can jeopardize the success of a change initiative. Among the reasons for resistance are:

- Fear of the unknown
- Perceived threat to the status quo
- Perceived threat to image or professional identity
- Potential threat to a personal or power base
- Fear of not being able to do the work that may be required (fear of failure)
- Fear of being exposed as incompetent
- Intentional malfeasance!

In his book, *Beyond the Wall of Resistance* (1996), Rick Maurer, a highly regarded expert in the field of organizational change and resistance, defines resistance as "a force that slows or stops movement" (p. 23). Engaging in or resisting change involves an investment of energy, which for many is a precious commodity and depleted personal resource. Fortunately the energy required to resist change also has the potential to convert to energy that supports change. Nurse managers are catalysts for that conversion.

KNOW YOUR RESISTANCE HOT SPOTS

Many managers believe that negative comments are "bad" and staff silence and lack of complaining or feedback are "good." While both may be true, so is the opposite. Resistance wears many masks. Overt resistance generally includes what you see and hear, such as verbal protests, endless questions, sarcasm, and excuse making. Resistance becomes especially problematic when it becomes covert. Your nurse manager antenna will tell you, "Something is up," even though things look fine. You may hear staff grumblings but you can never pin down the source. Examples of covert, destructive, resistant behaviors include sabotage, such as not showing up for meetings, incomplete tasks related to the change initiative, and deliberate attacks on persons, processes, and equipment. Individuals and groups can demonstrate endless creative capacities to resist change.

Underlying both overt and covert resistance on its deepest level is usually an issue of fear of the unknown; perceived loss of status, power, and control; or self-doubt, either from a personal or group perspective. **Dealing with matters of resistance is never optional.** If you are aware that it exists, ignoring it will only give it strength. When nurse managers are informed and mindful of the dynamics of resistance, they acquire a distinct advantage for facilitating change.

THE 20/60/20 RULE OF RESISTANCE

This simple 20/60/20 Rule of Resistance provides an unscientific yet useful guide for determining the extent of resistance that may be present among your staff. Knowing these approximate percentages and using your nurse manager antenna will enable you to meet resistance and manage it before it gets out of hand.

The 20% Who Love Change

These individuals thrive in a changing workplace. They are your champions for change, your cheerleaders. These supporters never lose sight of the patient. They put actions behind their words and do what needs to be done. Some staff may consider these individuals to be weird or "possessed" by an unknown force. Because of their support they can be vulnerable to or held suspect by their peers as "sucking up to the boss."

The 60% Who Wait and See

When the subject of change is introduced, approximately 60% will sit politely, listen, and appear interested. What happens inside their heads is another matter. This 60% is probably thinking, "How is this change going to mess up my life?" They are neither supporting nor resisting. They quickly move into a mode of wait and see. They are mulling things over, need more time to see and believe why change is necessary, and may reserve endorsement or engagement until they are convinced. The good news is that in the end these 60% will merge with the enthusiastic 20% in accepting proposed change. This 80% now represents a critical mass that is ready to move forward with varying degrees of speed. What about the remaining 20%?

The 20% Who Take 80% of Your Time

Resistance within this group is particularly complex and difficult to manage because the behavior is generally covert in nature. In this situation, staff members wear their smiley-face masks that hide their true character: Freddy from *Nightmare on Elm Street*. Resistance can sound like support in statements such as, "That seems like a very good plan; you can count on me for support." Don't count on it! Conversely, some who say "That will never work!" may not be resistors. In fact, they may become your strongest supporters once they have a chance to express their reasons and seek clarification. When resistance occurs behind your back it can turn nasty and has the potential to cause extensive damage to your change management efforts and workplace relationships.

BEWARE THE WORKPLACE SABOTEUR

These most challenging resistors are the (thankfully) rare few who openly with other personnel (but behind your back) "trash" the proposed change, you, the workplace, and the organization. They have no intention of ever supporting the change and make it their mission to ensure that "it" will never happen. These people are not happy campers and will make sure no one else is either. They are especially adept in recruiting physicians to join "the resistance." These individuals are not poor misguided souls. They have forgotten their professional role, their standards and code of ethics. Instead they have chosen the role of professional saboteur who will challenge you to your greatest power struggle. They typically possess informal power and influence within the staff group, can undermine your authority, and are very difficult to catch in the act.

If you have someone like this on staff you may not know it. The night shift can be a hotbed for propagating resistance and recruiting members for "the movement," especially when staff are permanently assigned to this shift. Once you get wind that sabotage, bad-mouthing, or complaining to patients (and anyone else who will listen) exists, it must be dealt with. When patients become drawn into the fight or aware of staff dissatisfaction, it frightens them, compromises trust, and negatively affects care. The longer this behavior is allowed to continue, the greater will be the damage and some will be irreparable, causing staff to leave and patient care to suffer. The bottom line is, this behavior is inconsistent with professional standards and the code of ethics.

MANAGING RESISTANCE

So how do you deal with resistance? Watch for it, attempt to understand it, and fearlessly nip it in the bud! The following scenario describes a typical mild to moderate expression of resistance from staff:

> The stage is set. You are about to deliver an elegant soliloquy on impending change. All players are assembled and you begin. As you look about the audience you notice that some have discovered that their shoes are absolutely fascinating, others are gazing out the window, and one or two valiantly struggle to keep their eyes open while stifling a yawn that threatens to explode their lungs. Bravo! Your message delivery was Tony Award–worthy. Feeling confident and comfortable that you communicated the right message, to the right people, at the right time, you ask if there are any questions. The pause seems as interminable as Simon and Garfunkel's "The Sound of Silence" plays in your head. Finally some brave soul comments, "Sounds like a good idea to me." Music to your ears! Then a voice from the back mutters, "Been there, done that, bought the t-shirt," followed by a series of bobblehead nods from those sitting closest to the voice of resistance. You are startled into your own awkward silence.

You are face to face with the masked presence of resistance. This form of resistance is not your enemy. **In fact, it can be a healthy ally in the process of facilitating change and staff engagement.** The trick is to know the difference and that resistance at all levels can be managed.

DON'T BACK DOWN

Organizational change when not managed well can be a catalyst for arousing nurses' anger and a host of other negative responses. **Unresolved and mismanaged anger among nursing staff can lead to resistance toward change, poor quality of care, and disruption in quality of work life.** As nurse manager, it is vitally important to address staff anger. But many nurse managers are uncomfortable in managing this challenge, preferring to hide in their office instead. Here is one reassuring thought, although snarky comments (at a staff meeting) may sound inappropriate, the fact that they are spoken in front of you may signal that staff members feel safe enough to express themselves in your presence. On the other hand, they may be testing you to see how you will react. **When you hear cynicism, negativity, and nasty asides always assume that there is more behind those words.** It is your job to find out what lies below! If you ignore this behavior:

- It will not go away. It will probably get worse and take on a life of its own.
- It will feed and reinforce staff perception that "management doesn't care" or "they never listen to us anyway."
- It can create a "we" versus "them" mindset among staff.

How you respond will determine if the mask comes off and stays off. You can shut down communication with a response such as, "I'm just following orders." (Add drama by throwing your hands in the air!) This is guaranteed to leave staff feeling unsupported, angrier, or more frustrated. Or, you can welcome the remark as an opportunity to open a door to exploration, learning, and mutual growth. When you are *seen* to be comfortable at managing resistance, you inspire confidence and the feeling that "we're in this together."

FAST FACTS in a NUTSHELL

- Resistance creates opportunities for conversations and personal growth.
- Facilitating meaningful conversations in the presence of resistance is a bit like peeling an onion. Be prepared for multiple layers and occasional tears. The end is worth it.

HANDLING CYNICS AND NAYSAYERS

The following dialogue suggests one way to respond to a comment such as, "Here we go again, another flavor of the month initiative!"

You can either respond immediately or take some time to think about what you need to say. Sometimes it is helpful to ask staff to hold their comments until after the presentation when there will be opportunities for feedback. Or you can stop your presentation and respond to questions and comments. Each staff and situation is different and you will have to determine what works best for you.

Take a breath. Acknowledge the person and say, "What you have to say is important to me. I am hearing that you believe this proposed change is not new and that you don't seem happy with how things went before. I would like to hear more about your experience." Continue using your Communication 101 skills. When you interact with staff in this manner, you are modeling effective relationship principles and competencies and meeting a basic human need to be treated with dignity and respect. This is nursing practice's therapeutic relationship in action! The following list summarizes the potential benefits from this type of healthy conversation:

- **Demonstrates support for staff.** It tells staff you are listening, willing to take time to hear what they say and to validate their presence at the meeting.
- **Demonstrates that you can handle criticism.** It tells staff that it is safe for them to express themselves.
- **Engages staff in meaningful dialogue.** Asking open-ended questions invites two-way conversations.
- **Builds trust.** At a time when cynicism is rampant and trust in leaders and their decisions can be very low, this approach can build or restore trust.
- **Helps you determine the level of resistance among staff.** Sarcastic, cynical and abrasive remarks are the "tip of the iceberg." Pay attention to body language. Behaviors such as folded arms, crossed legs, and eyes rolling backward may be cues that staff members are disengaging and require follow-up.
- **Creates an opportunity for you to assess the quality of your communication.** It is important to reflect on the quality of your message, its delivery, your body language, staff response, and its impact as staff members leave the meeting.
- **Demonstrates empathy.** When you convey empathy to staff, you reinforce the need for nurses to extend empathy to one another as implied in professional standards of practice.
- **Creates opportunities to listen for what is not being said.** Only 7% of communication is verbal. What is the message beneath the words? It is your job to find out.

- **Helps staff name their feelings.** Nurses often struggle with naming what they are *feeling* because of previous learning.
- **Helps staff learn how to manage their feelings.** Conversations about resources to help staff members manage stress are helpful even though they may be reluctant to admit that they need it.
- **Facilitates dialogue about what staff members are doing well, what they are proud of, and what they can do better.** Staff can easily get bogged down in the muck and the mire of change. You must create the momentum to keep staff moving forward. Try saying something like "That was then, this is now, and the decisions have been made. Our challenge is to make this happen. We will monitor the process, evaluate outcomes, and make revisions or recommendations."
- **Clarifies information about decision making: what is negotiable, and what is not.** Many staff members do not understand who has accountability and authority for what aspects of decision making. Explaining their roles in the decision-making process clarifies where their input is welcome. This minimizes their frustration when they voice their opinions, expect actions to be taken, and receive a less-than enthusiastic response.

FAST FACTS in a NUTSHELL

Summary

- Listening and responding to what is not being said is a powerful tool for self-discovery for you and your staff.
- When all else fails: If you can't change the people, change the people!

REFERENCE

Maurer, R. (1996). *Beyond the wall of resistance.* Austin, TX: Bard.

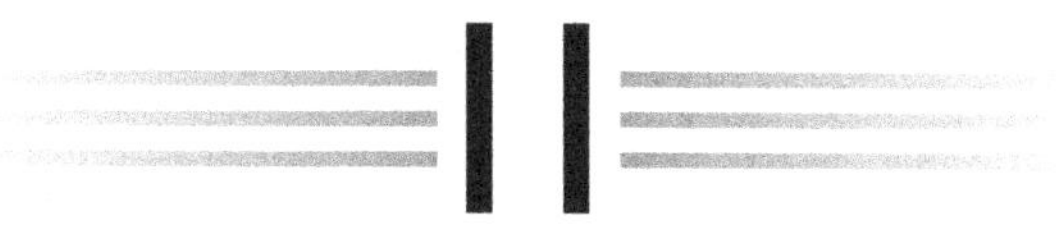

Got Attitude?

Managing the Good, the Okay, and the Downright Ugly!

It is an interesting fact of work life that many staff members believe their attitude at work is the fault of someone or something outside themselves. As a nurse manager one of your greatest challenges is to manage attitude in the workplace. This chapter introduces the concept of attitude, discusses the power it can have on the quality of care, work life, and workplace relationships, and provides tips for influencing positive change.

In this chapter, you will learn:

1. The impact of attitude in the workplace
2. The 35/55/10 Attitude Scale: the good, the okay, and the downright ugly!
3. Basic strategies for managing attitude

WORKPLACE ATTITUDE: GOT SOME?

Attitude (with a capital A) in today's workers is pandemic and is best summed up by Antonio, a character from the popular 1990s sitcom *Wings*, who said, "Gaze fondly upon today for tomorrow is bound to suck worse!" Negative attitudes may be a by-product of change in the workplace and reflect what is really happening at a deeper level with respect to staff's feelings, perceptions, and behaviors. **Most often, such attitudes emanate from feelings of low self-esteem, powerlessness, low level of trust, a sense of betrayal, disrespect, mental and physical exhaustion, and mismanagement.** More recently, compassion fatigue has surfaced as potential cause for negativity at work.

Attitude is a choice. Regardless of our circumstances at work **each of us has the power to choose our attitude**. The only time we are not held responsible for our attitude is if we are psychotic—and there are medications to treat that! The ability to thrive in a changing workplace largely depends on the attitude staff members choose in response to what is going on in each individual's internal and external environment.

THE 35/55/10 ATTITUDE SCALE (THE GOOD, THE OKAY, AND THE DOWNRIGHT UGLY)

Change comes in the form of a staff attitude menu with choices that include the good to great, the okay and so-so, and the downright ugly. The percentage breakdown on the Attitude Scale: 35/55/10. Although unscientific, this schematic works well a gauge for measuring potential staff attitudes! The numbers reinforce the fact that most of your staff, when led by excellence, will eventually manage whatever changes come their way. But a few never will and they may give you more than one sleepless night.

The 35% With Good-to-Great Attitudes

Nurses working part-time, in community settings, or in 9-to-5 practice settings appear to be the happiest of all. They readily admit that they can "Come to work, do my job, and at the end of my shift leave the politics behind, and feel good about what I've accomplished." Many other nurses actively avoid getting caught up in the gossip and backbiting, and are able focus on patient care. They skilfully manage peer relationships and try to "get along with everyone." When they find themselves in uncomfortable situations (e.g., gossip, bullying, or compromised practice), they will do the right thing. These nurses are your role models for demonstrating healthy workplace relationships and meeting practice standards. Your recognition and support is vital to keeping them motivated and engaged in their practice. Be mindful of the optics of recognizing these staff, as their colleagues with negative attitudes may perceive your behavior as favoritism. They can then target the individuals as "teacher's pets" and make work life difficult for these nurses who are just trying to do their jobs.

THE 55% WITH OKAY-TO-SO-SO ATTITUDES

When change initiatives are ramping up, pressure on you and staff increases in various ways, staffing is generally tight, and most staff members are in survival mode. There may be evidence that application of the professional standards of practice is weakening. Professional nursing care is at risk of becoming task focussed and routine oriented. Patient/client-centered care, continuity of care, and nursing care plans may also become casualties. The consequence of all these stressors is potential violation of practice standards through omission, placing nurses' licenses on the line.

At a time like this, nurses are vulnerable to the negative attitudes of a few, but powerful staff. When negativity abounds, most staff cope by trying to "go with the flow" to avoid trouble or causing problems. This survival strategy can lead to their unwitting participation in creating toxic workplaces. For example, when there is bullying in the workplace, individuals who are not directly involved know what is happening but say nothing for fear of rocking the boat or risking the wrath of the bully. In adopting this stance they become bystanders and accomplices in the bullying process.

When nurses experience negative attitudes and behaviors among their colleagues, they often feel that they should do or say something. However, they may be reluctant to do so for fear of disrupting the relationships on which they regularly depend. Others feel unsure about what to say or how to handle negative and toxic situations. They rarely realize that the negative attitudes also have an impact on the quality of patient care by impairing communication between team members. Although staff may be vulnerable to negative influences at this time, they are equally open to positive ones. This is particularly true when nurse mangers deal with unacceptable behavior and create opportunities for staff to talk about what respectful, accountable, and professional attitudes and behaviors look like.

The 10% With Downright Ugly Attitudes

Some staff have a high need for order, predictability, and control. They prefer to follow specific routines, work with their chosen group of individuals, and take breaks at the same time no matter what. Organizational change can pose a huge threat to those who require stable environments. No matter how many explanations or how much time they have had to digest the change process, they will never accept what is going on. They will not change! Nurse managers will spend an inordinate amount of time trying to convince, cajole, and influence their behavior. It will not work! They see no role for themselves in helping create stability; they believe that it is the manager's and everyone else's job to "fix it."

MISERY LOVES COMPANY

Staff with miserable attitudes need company to fuel their fire and are expert at recruiting a following. Their attitude often reflects pride in holding steadfast to the "old ways," refusing to accept change, and seeing themselves as purists (real nurses who may actually resurrect their old nurse's cap for added effect). They do their best work behind the scenes, when the nurse manager is out of sight. In many instances they are seen, especially by physicians, as the stars of the workplace, the "terrific nurses"—the epitome of efficiency and excellence. That is debatable.

A TOUGH CHALLENGE

Despite the fact that they do not support the direction in which the practice setting is heading, those with ugly attitudes often refuse to leave or transfer. The hang on, convinced that "things will get back to normal." Some have very little insight into how their attitude is affecting their colleagues or patient care. Others, who are close to retirement, may have a sense of entitlement and believe that their attitude is not a problem: It is "just the way I am." When this attitude prevails, other staff members learn to work or "pussyfoot" around them and will even defend or make excuses for their behavior.

Downright ugly behaviors present nurse managers with huge personal and professional challenges that can test the manager to the point where he or she may want to leave! In the end, however, after being managed from a performance perspective, some staff with toxic behaviors may have to leave. They lack either the self-awareness or the desire to improve their attitude. If these individuals are not managed, they along with their cohorts will ultimately threaten the quality of care and the ability of other staff to thrive. *Caution:* Challenging a particular staff member's attitude is one of the most difficult performance management issues and must be managed carefully with lots of documentation; time for remedial action; alignment with the standards of practice, code of ethics, and organizational values; and a high degree of courage and confidence on your part.

FAST FACTS in a NUTSHELL

- Message to staff: Attitude is a choice. Choose wisely.
- Message to self: I cannot be responsible for changing staff's attitudes. I can only create the conditions and hope this helps individuals to reflect and choose an attitude that helps them to thrive.

THE BOTTOM LINE

Staff members are responsible for the attitude they choose. When they choose behaviors that reflect toxic attitudes, they must be held accountable within the context of their standards of practice. Nurse managers are ultimately responsible and accountable for ensuring that staff behaviors are consistent with professionalism in practice. Managing negative attitudes is difficult and uncomfortable but essential, for your sake and that of your staff. Quality care and healthy interpersonal relationships will not happen without attention to this component.

PROFILING CLASSIC UGLY ATTITUDES AMONG A GROUP OF CHARACTERS

Toxic characters are typically found in most workplaces. They create strain on workplace relationships and detract from patient care. The three types that follow demonstrate classic ugly attitudes, but there are many more out there. The degree of distress these characters cause is generally mild to moderate. As their manager, count yourself among the fortunate if you have only one of these characters on staff. In many settings all three are present.

"Negaholics"

What They Do

These individuals are chronically negative. They are predisposed to whine and complain about everything, and anything that breathes is an audience. Nothing is ever good enough and no amount of jumping through hoops to please them or brighten their mood will put a smile on their faces. For example, as the new shift comes on duty, the negaholics will greet them with, "We had a rough night and you are going to have a terrible day! Bye!"

Another favorite behavior is repetitious nattering about the same issue. When asked what they plan to do about the situation, the response is usually silence and glazed eyes. Or they will say, "I don't know, it's not my job to figure it out." Whining and complaining can be a symptom of an unexpressed feeling or need. The problem is that other staff members admit that the negaholics have the power to propel them into a negative mindset and turn a day they were looking forward to into a nightmare.

What They May Want

Attention, recognition, personal power, or help.

What They Don't Want

To do anything to improve the situation.

What You Can Do

- Try to identify what they are *not* saying.
- Listen more than you speak (but not forever).
- Do not under any circumstance become their psychotherapist!
- Be careful about how you offer help. When you ask, "How can I help you?" (to correct your bad behavior), the unspoken message is, "You may not be capable of helping yourself; therefore you need me to help you." When you take responsibility for the behavior of staff members, you take away their power to help themselves. They then have an excuse to defer their responsibility; it gets them off the hook. Instead, point out their behavior and ask them how it could affect quality of care and their peer relationships. Point out that this behavior is inconsistent with a professional practice environment, and ask what they think they can do to improve their behavior. Help them to develop a time-specific plan for managing their behavior. Express confidence in their ability to create a positive outcome.
- Engage all staff in conversations about behaviors that strengthen workplace relationships and ones do not. Reinforce your expectations regarding professional conduct of all staff.
- Be prepared to go down the performance-management road if chronic negativity persists.

Rumor and Gossip Mongers

What They Do

These staff members have the dirt on everyone and love to share what they know with anyone who will listen. The research community has only recently weighed in on the benefits of workplace gossip. Some researchers contend that "good gossip" is a positive relational tool used predominantly among women to strengthen connectedness. However, in some workplaces, staff members describe the hurtful effects of gossip because it threatens harmony. They also express discomfort when approached by someone with a "juicy bit about someone else." Once again, individuals are inclined to respond with silence for fear of compromising their relationships or because they do not know how to manage the behavior.

What You Can Do

- Ask yourself why individuals keep hurtful gossip alive and well, even though most would like it to stop.
- Ask staff what gossip does for them and what it may be masking.
- Recognize that gossip is a complex behavior that may relate to power and control issues in the workplace.
- Ask yourself and staff, "What situations in the workplace lead us to feel powerless?"
- Help staff to look at and name the situations that create feelings of powerlessness, and facilitate discussion about how to handle the situations differently.
- Invite further conversations about how staff can strengthen positive personal and professional power.

"Houseplants"

What They Do

These individuals have an incredible knack for doing as little as possible. They sit on a chair for most of the shift, managing to avoid answering call bells, the telephone, or inquiries. Everyone knows their game, yet few to none will ever say anything. Meanwhile staff resentment builds. If a staff member makes a comment, it is usually humorous and ultimately futile. Houseplants are expert at ignoring dirty looks and subtle rebukes. Staff feel that they are doing the houseplant's work in addition to their own and will wonder why the manager is not doing anything about this individual at a time when staffing is tight and every pair of hands needed.

Sometimes houseplants are worn out and unaware that they are not doing their share of the work. Sometimes they are lazy! When they lack the insight and feel unable to do the work they were hired to do, they are not living up to the requirements of their professional contract. If there is a medical reason, nurse managers must help these staff come to the realization that they may require medical attention. If their behavior is linked to attitude, your challenge is greater. It becomes a performance issue that cannot be ignored. In addressing the situation head on, you provide welcome relief for the staff member who is not sharing the load and his or her peers who are angrier than hornets! A win–win situation develops for all.

What You Can Do

- Be there! If you are not, you cannot know what is really going on.
- Periodically cruise through your workplace and observe the "flow" of activity to see who is doing what, who is with the patients, and who is sitting behind the desk.
- Look for patterns of activity among staff (e.g., who responds to call bells, phone calls, etc.).
- If you suspect houseplants in your midst, it is your job to uproot them!
- Meet with the underperforming staff member to point out your observations, the practice implications, and the impact on the team, and listen for his or her explanation. Ask about his or her plan to remedy the situation.
- State your expectations for improved performance and schedule a follow-up meeting.

FAST FACTS in a NUTSHELL

Summary

- Managing attitudes is essential for creating healthy workplace relationships.
- Healthy workplace relationships grow happy staff.
- Happy staff stays.

12

Got Queens, Princesses, and Workplace Terrorists?

Managing Their Reign of Terror

"Queen" behavior in the workplace is not unique to nursing. However, in a predominantly female workplace, anger, powerlessness, frustration, and feelings of disrespect exist. Such conditions can foster the emergence of particularly aggressive behaviors attributed to the presence of a workplace queen. This chapter describes one of the most toxic workplace behaviors and its serious impact on patient care, staff relationships, and quality of work life. Managing the overt and covert operations of workplace terrorist behavior are revealed.

In this chapter, you will learn:

1. To identify toxic behaviors in the practice setting
2. Tips for dethroning workplace queens and managing a toxic practice setting

WORKPLACE TERRORISM UNCOVERED

The use of the terms *terror* and *terrorism* in the context of workplace behavior may seem extreme, but the impact of toxic behaviors can be devastating to individuals, demoralizing to entire staffs, and damaging to the reputations of organizations and, tragically, patient care. The good news is that, thankfully, only a very small percentage of staff ever earn to title of the "queen" of workplace terrorism. Many queens seem unaware of their toxic behavior or status while almost everyone else is acutely aware. Queens are tough to manage (especially in a unionized environment). Many nurse managers can become victims of a queen when engaged in a power struggle. In a few of the worst-case scenarios, queens and their princesses deliberately set out to "destroy" any nurse manager who gets in their way, and the rate of turnover of nurse managers in a toxic practice setting becomes the lore of legends. Battles against a manager can be so psychologically fierce and physically draining that managers are unable to do their jobs and eventually end up leaving rather than continue the struggle. This situation is particularly distressing when it occurs (not exclusively) within the environment of professional caring.

Workplace queens are the embodiment of unprofessional behavior that is nothing short of bullying. Although the topic of bullying is discussed in Chapter 13, queens deserve their own chapter because of their looming presence, prominence, and ability to survive for decades within the culture of nursing. Most nurses encounter a queen at least once in their career. They are well versed in insisting how "things are done around here." For this reason, they are frequently feared and revered at the same time. Their power is insidious and they do their best work and their most damage where and when detection is least likely.

The impact of the queen's toxicity is not limited to the practice setting and can leech into other areas of the organization, community, and beyond.

AN OVERVIEW OF KINGS AND QUEENS

The counterparts of queens and princesses are, of course, kings and princes. The presence of a queen/king and his or her followers can seriously undermine efforts to recruit and retain. In nursing, there are likely to be more queens than kings because of the larger number of women in the profession. Although this chapter focuses on queens and princesses, it does not mean that men are exempt from similarly poor conduct.

Gender usually determines how toxic behaviors play out in the workplace. Research on women's patterns of relating, managing anger, and bullying provides valuable insight into the queen's behavior. The culture of nursing is ripe for queen behavior, as evident in the old nursing old adage, "Everyone knows we eat our young," which has lingered far too long. Workplace queens thrive because of nurses' proclivity for stabilizing relationships. Not wanting to cause trouble, nurses maintain a culture of silence and apparent calm on the surface, while just beneath all hell breaks loose. Queens exist because they can. This tacit acceptance of queens and fear of dealing with them must end if nursing is to retain and recruit staff. Although tongue-in-cheek humor is used to bring this subject into the light of day, queen behavior is no laughing matter. "You can't change what you don't acknowledge," to quote Dr. Phil, and nursing must take a long hard look at a profession that permits staff members to hurt one another while proclaiming they are "caring" professionals. The practice must end through reflection, examination, education, meaningful change and yes, disciplinary action for conduct unbecoming to a nurse.

QUEENS AND THEIR COURTIERS

Queens have such great power in the workplace that it often allows them to supplant the role and authority of the nurse manager. Their power source comes from their ability to create a following in the workplace, inspire loyalty, and engage other staff in actions contravening healthy team relationships. The queen's followers, or "queens in training," often mimic the behaviors of the queen but generally do not possess the same degree of power.

FAST FACTS in a NUTSHELL

- The toxic impact of queen behavior is compounded when others are called to their majesty's court.
- Some go willingly while others join out of fear of becoming the next target.

Queens and princesses employ a number of tactics to maintain their position and power. Without the benefit of psychoanalysis, it is difficult to speculate on their motivation. Why do individuals who profess to be caring resort to soul-destroying behavior? Some say it is typical of oppressed group behavior, while others conclude that it is misplaced or misdirected anger. There are many theories as to why queen behavior exists. What is puzzling is the fact that it has been allowed to persist in direct contrast to standards of practice and has been tolerated by nurse leaders who are accountable for promoting harmonious workplace relationships. Most troubling is the naïve thinking that assumes queens limit their behaviors to their peers. In the name of patient care, this must be challenged by nurse managers, The following examples illustrate a few of the preferred tactics of queens and princesses, and the chapter on bullying will enlighten you even more.

Intimidation: The Queen Is Not Amused!

A typical scenario becomes a regular routine of the queen or princess and plays out as follows:

> A staff nurse returns from break and is met by the icy stare of the queen, who stands in the hallway staring at her watch, then glaring at the nurse, then back at her watch, and then back to the nurse. She is silent as she delivers the final "if looks could kill" nonverbal blow! Without speaking the queen has accomplished an act of intimidation designed to make the nurse feel any number of emotions, including:

- Guilt—for being perceived as late when he or she probably was not
- Fear—of being watched
- Anger—at being embarrassed in front of others
- Resentment—at being treated as a child
- Anxiety—about what may happen next

Over time, these negative emotions build up inside individuals and groups. If not managed, they create secondary issues, including illness, avoidance, and breakdowns in communication that impair team functioning and patient care. To prevent repeated victimization, the targeted nurse may call in sick, change his or her clinical assignments, and keep communication to a bare minimum.

Blaming Others: Off With Their Heads!

Queens have a knack for blaming others and rarely accept responsibility for their own behavior. Nothing is ever the fault of the queen. If you are waiting for insight to occur, it may never happen. Despite great efforts to help, some staff never accept responsibility for their actions.

Ridiculing Others: Peasants Be Gone!

A favorite tactic is to use an imperious tone of voice with young graduates. The goal is to disempower and humiliate a nurse novice with a remark such as, "You don't know that? Everyone knows that!" Or, "What *did* they teach you in school anyway?"

Disappearing Others: You See Me, but I Choose to Not See You!

In the presence of the queen and princesses, the victim is treated as invisible. For example, if a nurse on the target list walks into a room where the queen and princesses are holding court, the nurse is completely ignored. The queen makes no eye contact whatsoever and avoids directing any remarks to the individual or acknowledging his or her presence.

PUBLIC FLOGGINGS: A POWER-BOOSTING MOMENT!

Being told "That's stupid!" or "Don't be ridiculous!" diminishes self-worth and self-confidence. This behavior may eventually shut some people down to the point where they are filled with doubt about their ability to do their job, begin to question their judgment, and could become ill.

Exclusionary: So You Are Not on My "A" List? Too Bad, So Sad!

Certain staff may be deliberately excluded from social occasions. The buzz intensifies as courtiers speculate about why? Another common tactic is to inform new staff not to use specific rooms, equipment, or chairs until they come off the "probationary period."

DETHRONING WORKPLACE KINGS AND QUEENS

Managing queen behavior is never optional. How it is managed depends on the type of behavior, circumstances, experience of the manager, and resources available to support the process.

Queen behavior will not thrive in practice environments where:

- The nurse manager is present, not tucked away in an office.
- There is a requirement for adherence to nursing practice standards.
- Nurse managers possesses self-awareness and strong leadership skills.
- The focus is on patient/client-centered care.
- There are opportunities for staff development.
- Respectful behavior in the workplace is required.
- Staff members receive regular performance feedback.
- There are consequences for untoward actions.

FAST FACTS in a NUTSHELL

- Dethroning workplace queens and kings is never optional.
- Declare the buffet closed by saying, "Nurses will no longer eat their young!"

SPECIAL OPS TACTICS FOR NURSE MANAGERS

To tackle queen behavior in your workplace use both short-term and long-term strategies.

Short-Term Strategies

1. First, take care of yourself: Conduct a self-assessment (your readiness to deal with a very tough problem).
2. Write down what you know about the behavior. Determine the level of impact and develop a plan.
3. Schedule a meeting with the queen to discuss the issue(s). Be prepared for a sick call or excuse and the potential for endless delays. Avoid allowing this ploy to drag on (the queen's strategy is to wait you out).
4. Conduct the first meeting as per your performance management protocols. Point out the inappropriate behaviors. Identify your expectations for future conduct.
5. Link the queen's behaviors to the standards of practice that govern professional relationships and accountability.
6. Keep the meeting short (no more than 20 minutes)—this coveys a message that you are in charge)—preferably holding it in your office. After all, territoriality is a big issue in power struggles.
7. Express your confidence that the behavior will change and schedule check-in meetings.
8. Expect a sick call or a doctor's note identifying a need for short-term or long-term sick leave. Stay on top of the situation and modify your plan accordingly.

Long-Term Strategies

1. Schedule lunch-and-learn sessions or staff meetings that include conversations about the following:
   - Living the value of respect in our workplace
   - Bullying in the workplace
   - Accountability in healthy workplace relationships
   - Having difficult conversations
   - Standards of practice and code of ethics
2. Consult with other nurse managers about their approach to managing queen behaviors.
3. Discuss professionalism in practice.
4. Create opportunities for assertiveness training.
5. Consult with other departments about strategies to prevent and manage this type of behavior across the organization.

6. Review the effectiveness of managing untoward staff behaviors within the context of the organization's mission, vision, and values.

FAST FACTS in a NUTSHELL

Summary

- Queen behavior is not exclusive to nursing.
- Queens thrive because they can.
- Terrorism in the workplace cannot thrive when there is strong, effective leadership in a practice setting driven by the standards of professional practice.

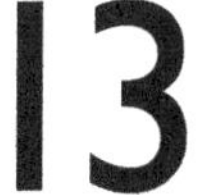

Got Bullying?

Managing the Sound of Silence

The phenomenon of bullying in nursing is not new. Yet despite policies of zero tolerance, bullying continues as an "organizational undiscussable" (Beer & Eisenstat, 2000) that incubates and proliferates in a culture of silence. Dealing with a workplace bully who is a nurse presents the nurse manager with time-consuming and extraordinary personal and professional challenges. This chapter focuses less on the troubling characteristics of bullies and more on what to do about them. The intent is to encourage you to take the necessary steps to fuel and support your resolve to rid your workplace of bullying behaviors.

In this chapter, you will learn:

1. Bullying is preventable
2. Your vital role in eliminating bullying from the practice setting
3. Skills and processes for managing bullying

THE BEGINNING OF THE END OF WORKPLACE BULLYING IN NURSING

In the 1990s, bullying in the workplace was acknowledged through the introduction of Zero Tolerance policies in many organizations.

Although its presence was acknowledged with the introduction of these policies, it was rarely talked about openly. Nurse managers and staff remain reluctant or unsure as to how to characterize or manage this behavior. Many managers who attempt to deal with this issue continue to struggle to receive organizational support, and the process intensifies when the union becomes involved. The presence of a bully is still tolerated in silence, and victimized staff members continue to leave "to further advance" their careers. Remaining staff tiptoe around the bully, excusing his or her actions with, "You get used to it," or "They don't really mean anything by it. She (or he) is a really good nurse." Even with the assistance of the evolving and enlightened support of human resource staff, bullying continues to flourish. **The fact that bullying is still prevalent speaks to the issue that current strategies are not working.**

Nurses continue to turn on one another, especially during significant organizational change and deteriorating workplace conditions that evoke feelings of powerlessness, fear of the unknown, and frustration. As daunting as it may seem, nurse managers have the greatest ability to end bullying in clinical practice settings.

MONKEY IN THE MIDDLE

In unionized environments, nurse managers can be set up for a "monkey in the middle" situation. They become caught between the perpetually warring factions of union and management, where what began as an issue of negative behavior of a staff member becomes an attack on the manager's credibility.

ARE YOU UP FOR THE CHALLENGE?

Before dealing with a bully, many nurse managers will quietly ask themselves if they are "up for this." Some believe that they may be "hung out to dry" and will search their souls asking if sacrificing their mental health is too high a price to pay. Some may ask if the situation is really all that bad. Others may suppose that if they did not witness the behavior, they cannot do anything about it. A few may even excuse the behavior or justify it by noting, "Well, that's just the way they are." The cost of inaction is high, and patients and staff will pay the price. Staff will lose respect for their manager, thinking (sometimes rightfully so) that nothing is being done. They will continue to live and work in a state of fear, and deep inside you will know that you are not doing the right thing. In the end, good staff will be left to manage a struggle that should not be theirs in the first place, and the bully will retain the seat of power above all.

Patient care suffers chiefly due to failure of effective communication between the victim and the bully borne from the fear of criticism or ridicule by the bully, or both. This situation can lead to oversight in care or unreported clinical information, and becomes a practice issue that violates standards of practice standards.

WHY BULLIES THRIVE

Despite our knowing a great deal about workplace bullies—what makes them tick, their impact on victims, peers and quality of care, and costs to the organization—bullying continues. Why? Because it can! It remains grossly underreported and unmanaged and rarely is brought to the attention of the professional regulatory body. Bullies thrive on silence. We tolerate bullying behavior because of:

- **Fear**: Bullies are scary! Many nurse managers are afraid of bullies.
- **Denial**: Managers may deny the existence of a bully in *their* workplace.
- **Organizational nonsupport**: There may be a lack of meaningful policies or support for nurse managers.
- **Exhaustion:** Managers may lack the stamina or time to go down that long and winding road of performance management.
- **Escalation:** There may be a (legitimate) concern that the behavior will escalate into physical violence, at or outside of work.
- **Unwillingness to take on the union**: The possibility of an adversarial encounter with the union or litigious actions by the staff member is not something most managers want to take on.
- **Costs**: Managers may be reluctant to hop on the medical leave of absence merry-go-round, which occurs when the bully, realizing the toxic behavior is no longer acceptable, takes medically approved sick leave, comes back, goes off again, and returns ad infinitum—sometimes for years!
- **Workload**: Managers may dread the consequences of adding more difficult work to their already heavy workload.
- **Credibility**: Managers may worry that the tables will be turned and he or she will be seen as the real problem.

- **Reluctance**: Even with support it is something most organizations do not want to tackle.

NOT FOR THE FAINT OF HEART

Given the personal energy crisis that most of us are experiencing in today's workplaces, many nurse managers shake their heads in despair at the thought of a staff member who bullies. Many will wearily declare, "I don't have the time or the energy for this." Not having the time is not an option. The implications of not managing bullying behavior are far-reaching and include:

1. **The obvious**
   - Staff will leave.
   - Care will suffer.
   - Sick time will increase.
   - Morale will tank.
   - Bullies hold onto their power.
2. **The less obvious**
   - Bullying *is* unprofessional conduct.
   - Managers cannot (by virtue of their legislation and standards of practice) turn a blind eye to unprofessional conduct.
   - Bullying violates standards of practice and is unethical according to nurses' code of ethics.
   - You are leading a workplace that may be driven by fear (generated by the bully).
   - This 1% (the bully) of your staff is holding at least 99% psychologically hostage!
   - You will lose the respect of your staff.
   - The word on the street will be, "Don't work there."

FAST FACTS in a NUTSHELL

- The underlying reason we tolerate bullying is fear.
- Nurse managers hold the most power organizationally and professionally to manage bullying behavior.
- Because nurse managers are ultimately accountable for managing bullying in the workplace, they must find the courage to manage their own and staff members' fear.

THE "SECRET" TO FINDING COURAGE

The secret is to adopt the attitude, "It's not personal; it's professional." Your leadership is required to ensure that patients receive nursing care delivered by competent professionals in a healing and safe practice environment. Your job is to ensure that this happens. There is no compromising when your standards require you to take action!

PRACTICE STANDARDS MATTER

When workplace bullies run amok, professional nursing practice becomes embroiled in and distracted by unhealthy and destructive relationships. In managing bullying behavior nurse managers send the following messages:

- As nurses we are duty and legally bound by our standards of practice to protect our patients and support our colleagues.
- Each registered nurse is accountable for his or her practice.
- Untoward behavior (unprofessional conduct) is inconsistent with professional conduct.

According to practice standards for nurse leaders, a key accountability is to ensure that staff complies with their practice standards. By linking bullying behavior to nursing practice standards, bullying becomes a noncompliant and unacceptable behavior. With full knowledge of the standards and their applications, the employment contract, appropriate organizational resources, and the right attitude and skill mix, nurse managers have the tools to eliminate bullying in the workplace.

A THREE-TIERED APPROACH FOR MANAGING BULLIES

Tier I: Self

Once you identify bullying behavior in your practice area, reflect on your feelings about the situation: Are you afraid of the bully? Does your workload leave you feel overwhelmed? Are you ready to take this on? Get a handle on your own situation before dealing with the bullying behavior.

If You Witness Bullying Behavior

- First, gather your thoughts and record observations, including dates and times.
- Plan your approach to meet with the bully, discuss the inconsistencies with expectations of professional practice, and identify consequences, articulate desired outcomes, establish parameters for improvement, and begin the process of implementing a remedial plan.
- Inform your boss and human resources (if appropriate) that you are about to tackle suspected bullying behavior, giving them a heads-up about your approach, your short-term and long-term plan, and your anticipated outcome.
- Seek support from a trusted colleague for practicing role playing in preparation for your conversation with the bully.
- Get a good night's sleep before the meeting.
- If the person (bully) has anger management issues, take this into consideration (e.g., you may want to leave the door slightly open, situate yourself closest to the door, or have a colleague nearby).
- Keep the meeting brief (15 to 20 minutes).

If You Are Aware of, but Have Not Witnessed, the Bullying Incident

- Don your Sherlock Holmes hat, perform your investigative homework, conduct a self-check, and begin the process of eliminating this destructive force.
- Assign priority status to managing this unprofessional conduct.
- Remind yourself that you must follow through with this action or staff morale and patient care will continue to suffer.
- Gather and record your facts: observations, time(s) and date(s) of incident(s), presence of others.
- Give a heads-up to the person to whom you report.
- Schedule an appointment with the staff.
- Before you meet, get a good night's sleep.
- Repeat the mantra, "It's not personal; it's professional."
- Develop a small support network or recruit a colleague to practice your feedback session before you meet with the staff person.
- Proceed according to performance management protocols.
- At the beginning of the meeting explain to the staff member that part of your professional administrative responsibility lies in overall accountability for the quality of care and work life

in this practice setting. This includes managing situations that may negatively influence patient care and staff relationships.
- Describe your observations, listen to feedback, and tell the person that you would like him or her to develop a plan for how to improve the behavior to meet practice standards.

Tier 2: Staff

- You have the administrative and professional accountability and responsibility for determining the impact of the behavior on staff and taking steps to reestablish harmony in the workplace. In doing so, you create a healing environment and a healthy workplace where people want to work. Of course you cannot discuss your intervention with staff.
- Most staff members know and hope you will deal with the workplace bully. The irony is that for obvious reasons of confidentiality, they will never know what steps you took to curb this individual's behavior. You can, however, send a subtle yet powerful message that healthy workplaces are mandatory for the provision of quality care and all staff members are accountable and responsible for their behavior at work.
- You can begin with a back-to-basics conversation about the non-negotiables with respect to professional practice, quality care, and healthy workplace relationships. This will be discussed at length in the chapters to follow. Staff will quietly be reassured about who is at the helm and appreciate that there is no place for fear in the workplace.
- Look for opportunities every day to connect standards with day-to-day care, relationships, and professional practice.

Tier 3: The Organization

- Raise the matter of zero tolerance at the leadership table to determine how extensive bullying is in the workplace, if it is being managed effectively and if not, why?
- Recommend a forum for other nurse managers to discuss the challenges of managing the "underbelly" of professional practice.
- Identify further organizational supports required to help nurse managers effectively manage bullying behavior.

Summary

- Managing bullying behavior is a professional responsibility and an act of courage. You can do both. You must!

REFERENCE

Beer, M., & Eisenstat, R. (2000). The silent killers of strategy implementation and learning. *Sloan Management Review, 41*(4), 29–40.

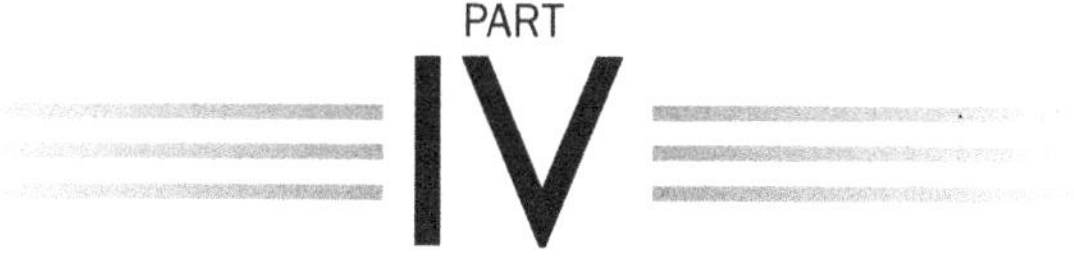

PART IV

Predicting Your Workplace Future

Create It! Manage It! Love It!

14

Mission Impossible?

Creating Work–Life Harmony

Recent research reveals that work–life balance—long considered an almost impossible goal—is, in fact, achievable, and that harmony at work and home can be obtained with the two complimenting one another. Nurse managers can play a significant role in facilitating harmony for themselves and staff by inspiring quality practice environments where staff well-being, healthy relationships, and professional practice creates tremendous satisfaction. At the end of the day, happy staff members are more likely to take this sense home with them. Creating a place where staff wants to work requires resolution of the tensions within nurses' deeply embedded work ethic of self-sacrifice that can also lead to disharmony. How do you lead by example to create quality workplaces? This chapter will help you to recognize the signs of disharmony and strategies for promoting a sense of well-being and harmony at work.

In this chapter, you will learn:

1. The impact of a "brushfire management" style on harmony at work
2. The necessity for engaging in personal change to course correct disharmony
3. Tips for completing your mission

THE PROBLEM

During the past decades when downsizing, restructuring and layoffs were the norm, nurse managers were catapulted into a maelstrom of leadership and operational situations that traditional styles of management could not resolve. In their struggle to adapt many nurse managers unwittingly adopted a "brushfire management" style that continues to this day. Although unlikely to be found in the management literature, this style is highly popular. Borne out of necessity, it is practiced on a daily basis with great intensity and is a major threat to quality practice environments.

Brushfire management occurs when busy managers are constantly trying to "put out fires." Days typically begin with a plan but within minutes of stepping into the practice environment, the demands begin and managers go from one crisis to another, responding to phone calls, knocks on doors, and a barrage of requests beginning with "Have you got a minute?" As a result, many managers feel mentally and physically exhausted by the end of the day, which frequently ends in the evening. A sense of inadequacy can develop, topped off with guilt about things left undone. If that were not enough, the situation replicates itself when the nurse manager goes home to meet the demands of family living and community membership.

REFLECTION: ARE YOU A "BRUSHFIRE MANAGER"?

You are if you demonstrate some of the following behaviors:

- Your wristwatch has 25 or more hours a day (sometimes you wear two watches).
- You feel stressed most or all of the time.
- You usually arrive at work with wet hair.
- You "can't get no satisfaction."
- You are related to Alice's White Rabbit and are frequently heard to mutter, "I'm late, I'm late, for a very important (meeting)."
- You have forgotten how to say "no."

- The papers scattered about your office because of a tornado last year (at least that is your story and you are sticking to it) are still there.
- You feel like a mouse running on a treadmill or a puppet on a string.
- Guilt is your new BFF (best friend forever)!
- You return to work after hours to "finish up"—or to fill a U-Haul with paperwork to take home.
- You carry two cell phones and use them both at the same time!

FAST FACTS in a NUTSHELL

- Harmony occurs when you are able to effectively manage your responsibilities at work, in your home, and in your community, leaving you with a sense of emotional and physical well-being.
- Effective management is not about being all things to all people.

A NOTE ABOUT "WHIRLING DERVISH SYNDROME"

If you are prone to a brushfire management style, you are at risk of succumbing to chronic "whirling dervish syndrome." Your symptoms may include:

- A sense of foreboding about never-ending challenges
- Vertigo, or feeling as if you are spinning in random circles
- The belief that you are going nowhere fast

Furthermore, you often walk backward finishing a conversation with one person as you head to a meeting. For managers with any of these symptoms or signs, burnout is a hair's breadth away.

If allowed to go unchecked, your physical and mental health may suffer, workplace relationships will deteriorate, and regret will be profound. And the question that begs an answer is, "Who will lead your staff if you are unable to lead yourself and personally demonstrate that sense of well-being at work and at home?"

WHEN BRUSHFIRE MANAGEMENT INTERFERES WITH YOUR PERSONAL LIFE

The following situations are all too common when work life creates disharmony in your personal life:

- You forget to pick your child up from piano lessons.
- You miss your daughter's soccer game.
- You take a leisurely bubble bath with your "Crackberry" to answer e-mails.
- You have no "me" time.
- Sex or sleep? You choose sleep.
- You are unable to participate in family events because you have "work to do."
- You allow "guilt" to follow you home from work.
- Your pets run for cover when you arrive home.
- You yell at your houseplants!

YOUR MISSION: TO SEEK AND ESTABLISH HARMONY WITHIN YOURSELF, AT WORK, AND AT HOME

Should you choose to accept it, **your mission is to embark on a journey of personal change**, to capture the essence of a state of well-being (harmony) within yourself, at home, and at work. When you do, you model a new way of being, professionalism at its finest, and leadership. Staff will be inspired to follow your lead.

In Accepting Your Mission

1. Know that if you keep doing what you've always done, you'll keep getting what you always got.
2. Engage in self-reflection to increase your understanding of why brushfire management has such a grip on you.
3. Be willing to engage in new learning.
4. Get comfortable with trying new ways of being, failing, and trying again.

If You Refuse to Accept This Mission

The risks of not accepting change puts you and your staff in survival mode as opposed to thriving mode. It places all of you on a slippery personal and professional slope. You also face the following dangers:

- Physical problems associated with not taking care of yourself may emerge.
- Emotional problems associated with pushing your feelings aside may erupt as you and staff struggle with multiple demands. When you fail to take time to reflect on your situation and feelings, you run the risk of increasing frustration, anger, resentment, and powerlessness that can lead to toxic attitudes and behaviors at work, inefficiencies in operations and care, and spillover into your personal life.
- Potential for increased staff absenteeism, high use of sick time, and an inability to recruit and retain staff are real possibilities when harmony at work is nonexistent.
- Complaints of "alienation of affection" from colleagues, family, and friends.

The best hope that you and staff have for achieving a sense of well-being and harmony is for you to go first!

FAST FACTS in a NUTSHELL

- The best way to achieve personal and professional work–life balance is to commit to change, take the lead in changing your behavior, and inspire staff to follow.
- In the short term, change is difficult; in the long term you may wonder, "Why did I wait so long?"

TIPS FOR COMPLETING YOUR MISSION

These tips work in all settings whether at home, at work, or in the community.

1. Take Care of Yourself First

You cannot effectively perform the role of nurse manager if you are suffering mentally, physically, and spiritually. Staff will take their cues from you and will experience any number of reactions in response to your signals. When you communicate well-being your staff's radar picks it up.

2. Just Say "No" (or a reasonable facsimile thereof, to escape charges of insubordination!)

Easier said than done. Sometimes we must question our motives. What are the benefits and consequences of saying "no"? Wise words from an unknown source advise, "Never do anything for someone else that they are perfectly capable of doing for themselves."

3. Reflect On and Realign Your Priorities

Is it essential that *you* do laundry every day? How is work distributed at home and at work? Does it really matter that your children do not mitre their corners when making their beds? What are the relationship costs of insisting that your home be on the Junior League Christmas at Home tour?

4. Nurture Your Relationships with Your Colleagues, Friends, and Family

When you find yourself caught up in brushfire management, it is easy to focus on the tasks and lose sight of the people in your life. As humans, we are vulnerable to taking others for granted until faced with the stunning reality that one day they may not be there when we really need them. Remember the old saying, "No one on their deathbed was ever thanked for staying late at the office."

5. Create "Me" Time

Creating "me" time is difficult for most of us. Women in particular are often guilt ridden if they take time away from perceived responsibilities. They view this as an act of selfishness. Family members question how they will survive when you are "off-limits." No matter what, resist the temptation to return to your old patterns of behavior. As in any other art form, the process of creating a new you takes practice and patience.

6. Actively Reduce the Number of Demands You Place on Yourself

"When all else fails, lower your standards" (source unknown). While you may shudder at the thought, think about this: In today's changing and complex workplaces, everyone is on a learning curve and super humans are still in the cloning phase.

7. Lighten Up

Laughter is good medicine. There is much in today's literature about the benefits of laughter, including similarity of the effects to that of meditation. Whether you are at home or at work, rediscovering your sense of humor and laughing out loud (releasing a flood of endorphins) becomes a powerful tool in achieving a sense of well-being. Within the culture of nursing "black" humor has played a significant therapeutic role in helping nurses manage stress and traumatic situations. Appropriate laughter at work psychologically lightens the load and can promote harmony. Use it or lose it!

8. Reframe Negative Situations

Look for opportunities and possibilities. Where there is crisis, there is opportunity. Focus on the art of the possible and the upside of negative situations.

9. Take a Technology Break

Leave your smart phone at home while on vacation. If your mind is at the office when you are on a beach, you are not in true vacation mode and are living a lie. Others will sense you are really not present. If the thought of being PD free causes palpitations, change is no longer optional: You need help!

10. Take Your Breaks (Including Vacations)

We know our bodies need rest, yet our nursing work ethic can get us into trouble, and soon we are beyond tired. Inadequate rest can cause manager to fall asleep at the computer's keypad and staff to fall asleep at the bedside, standing up! Patients must be thinking, "Here nurse, take my place!"

11. Take Bathroom Breaks

Many nurses claim to have the bladder of a camel. While attempting to make a joke, what they are not saying is they frequently do not "have time" to take a break. Managers should be mindful of the health implications of nurses placing their own physical needs behind patient care demands and remind staff about the importance of taking bathroom breaks.

12. Explore Alternative Therapies and Practices

The therapeutic benefits of mindfulness practice, meditation, therapeutic touch, Reiki, massage therapy, yoga, and reflexology can enhance our sense of harmony and well-being. These are but a few of the ways to de-stress and rebalance our minds and bodies. Anything that takes us away from work-related preoccupation is worth trying (wine will do it too, but is not recommended for this purpose).

13. Make Time for Physical Activity

Many nurses have a long way to go in learning how care for their minds, bodies and spirits. Most practitioners will admit that they are "too tired to exercise" at the end of a shift. Once again, guilt creeps in to remind us that we should know and do better. We also know physical activity of at least 30 minutes a day, five days, a week has tremendous health benefits and goes a long way in promoting a sense of well-being at work and at home.

14. Eat Properly

Giving staff a box of chocolates is not a Forrest Gump moment. Instead it becomes a feeding frenzy. Once again we know better, but a frenetic pace at work and shiftwork can lead to poor eating habits. Making time to eat healthy food regularly would be an important step forward on our learning curve toward wellness.

YOU: A WORK IN PROGRESS

Achieving a sense of well-being at work and at home is an individual, personal, and professional matter that can have serious implications if not addressed. Deciding to change and then inspiring change within and among your staff to achieve harmony will require a willingness and commitment to "try on new behaviors" aimed at creating a sense of well-being, enhancing performance, and creating healthier workplace relationships. If you have not done so already, start now by giving yourself permission to become a "work in progress" and see what unfolds. Invite staff to join you on your journey toward wellness. Call a meeting to discover what factors in your environment promote or inhibit an environment of wellness and quality of work life and determine what measures you can take to promote harmony amid chaos (the cynics will have a field day with this one, but do not let that stop you. The rest of staff will come up with great ideas). Periodically check in with staff to tell them how well you are doing and monitor their progress, create opportunities to exchange ideas, acknowledge and celebrate successes.

FAST FACTS in a NUTSHELL

Summary

- It is easy to talk about creating a place where people want to work and harmony exists. It is harder to "walk the talk" and create a workplace with a focus on wellness.
- Staff will watch your every move to see if you really mean what you say.
- For your own sake and the health of your staff, achieving a sense of well-being is not optional and you must go first!

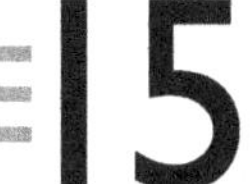

15 Creating Your Future

A Back-to-Basics Approach

Many nurse managers today, in addition to operational responsibilities, are accountable for promoting collaborative practice, demonstrating evidence-based practice, and incorporating research into their practice settings. To complicate things further, staffing is increasingly problematic and managers must now hire unregulated support staff to meet clinical demands. This situation adds a new layer of complexity to workplace relationships and work distribution. In this environment, it makes sense for nurse managers to create a solid plan, similar to a business plan, for mapping and creating their clinical future and how they will accomplish the work. Foundational to creating a clinical community of excellence is a clear statement of the practice setting's mission, vision, and values; promotion of trust; and an unshakeable belief about how everyone will work together. When these are present, staff thrives! A challenge, yes; impossible, no. Developing a back-to-basics action plan unifies staff and signifies strong nurse manager leadership. This chapter sounds an urgent call and provides a suggested path for nurse managers to do just that!

In this chapter, you will learn:

1. The importance of developing your practice setting's mission, vision, and values
2. The process for promoting trust and creating a team charter
3. The necessity of developing a back-to-basics plan as a step toward creating your future.

PREDICT YOUR WORKPLACE FUTURE: BEGIN BY CREATING YOUR MISSION, VISION, AND VALUES

Peter Drucker, an influential leader in management theory and practice, once said, "The best way to predict the future is to create it." What kind of workplace future do you want? What does staff want? These questions are normally not asked or answered by nurse managers and their staff. Instead, managers default to the organizational culture's formal statements about "our mission, vision, and values," which are typically generated by senior management during a strategic planning retreat.

WHEN STAFF LOOK BUT DO NOT SEE

Typically, nurse managers are expected to disseminate and discuss the organizational mission, vision, and value statements to secure buy-in to the future direction of the organization. Staff members respond, in turn, with cynical and tacit approval without ever truly owning the words or their intended message. The reason is that most staff has witnessed countless violations of newly minted organizational mission, vision, and values statements, stemming from no real plan as to how staff members will achieve these expectations.

The stories of leaders "not walking the talk" are legendary. **Too often, staff members experience fear in the workplace or are treated badly in organizations that simultaneously claim "people are our greatest assets."** They become disillusioned with these "organizational truths" and the mission vision, and values become meaningless.

FAST FACTS in a NUTSHELL

- Most staff members have a vague recollection that somewhere in their organization is a laminated plaque depicting the organizational mission, vision, and values statements. (It is usually doomed to suffer a lonely existence hanging between the elevators for everyone to see without really seeing.)

WHAT WE WANT—WHAT WE REALLY, REALLY WANT

Fundamentally, **most staff want and need to participate in meaningful work, contribute to the greater good, and know that they matter and make a difference in the lives of others.** When this happens, they are motivated to provide better care, achieve personal and professional success, and experience work life satisfaction. When units develop their own practice setting, mission, vision, and values that complement the larger organization's M, V, and V, they lay the foundation for creating their future. In the end, they feel a sense of ownership in the quality patient care outcomes and work life.

CREATING YOUR PRACTICE SETTINGS MISSION, VISION, AND VALUES

Especially during times of change, it is important for nurse managers to help staff reconnect to the meaning of their work and to the overall purpose of the organization. It is very easy for staff to feel disconnected at this time, to "go rogue," or do their own thing because "we've always done it this way."

FAST FACTS in a NUTSHELL

- Creating your practice setting's mission, vision, and values statements provide staff with a sense of direction, create context for the type of care/service delivered, and reinforce the moral and ethical drivers that guide the decisions and actions of the health care team.

- A **mission** describes the purpose of a clinical program or service and aligns staff on a shared journey.
- A **vision** reflects, ". . . our hopes for a preferred future" (Oakley & Krug, 1994, p. 227).
- **Values** represent the ethical and moral standards that will guide professional care and relationships in a practice setting.

WHERE TO START

1. Create opportunities to promote reflection and dialogue that provide staff with an opportunity to create their vision of how the members see themselves and the role they play in service delivery. Try asking the following questions, record the discussion, and use the answers in planning your vision statement.
   - Why do we exist as a practice setting? What is our shared purpose in the provision of health care service delivery? Why are we different?
   - Why is this service essential to overall organizational success? What business are we in? (Do not accept answers such as, "Because we care for mothers and children" or "Because we care for surgical patients.")
   - What special roles do our various team members play in the provision of care?
2. Reflect on and discuss the professional attributes and scopes of practice within all staff groups (nurses, care assistants, technicians, etc.).
3. Engage staff in the "Postcard from Home" exercise (see Appendix).
4. Conduct a values development exercise (see "Creating Our Values" in the Appendix).
5. Have a conversation about "Living Our Values" (see Appendix).
6. Have fun with the "Back to Our Future" exercise (see Appendix).
7. Use the "Back to the Future Follow-up Conversation Guide" to help staff identify specific suggestions for improving quality of work life or strengthening workplace relationships (see Appendix).
8. Review your mission, vision, and values annually to assess their effectiveness and determine whether they require modification.

BUILD TRUST AND THEY WILL COME

Trust building is the relational glue for effective interpersonal relationships. It determines how well staff members work together. Nurses know how to build and maintain trust within the context of the professional and therapeutic relationship to achieve successful patient/client care outcomes. Trust is equally important to team functioning. In many of today's chaotic and changing workplaces, trust at an interpersonal and organizational level is at an all-time low. Without trust in the manager, the practice setting metaphorically becomes a rudderless ship. Leaders require followers. **Without trust in staff members and their abilities, nurse managers cannot effectively lead.**

TRUST IN THE WORKPLACE

Trust is a complex and multilevel attribute. It encompasses integrity, honesty, transparency, and accountability, the essence of which is captured in nursing's standards of professional practice.

FAST FACTS in a NUTSHELL

- To thrive and manage in a changing workplace, nurse managers must be able to trust themselves, their staffs, their colleagues, and the organization.

Trust in Self

When relationships and work processes are muddied by constant change, organizational politics, and negative interpersonal relationships, trust in self is challenged. Under the constant scrutiny of staff's watchful eyes, **it is vital that nurse managers model trustworthy behavior and demonstrate trust in self.** Nurse managers who do what they say they will do, are transparent in their actions, authentic in their conversations, inspire confidence in staff ability to do the right thing, speak out on nurse's behalf on matters that affect clinical practice. These actions create environments of high trust.

Trust in Staff

Some nurse managers believe trust must be earned, while others believe that individuals are worthy of trust until they prove otherwise. Being willing to trust staff up front:

- Leaves the door open for mutual trust building
- Inspires accountability
- Implies that it is okay to take a leap of faith, try new things, and make appropriate independent decisions
- Creates a climate for developing future leaders

Trust in Colleagues

Changing workplaces may experience rapid turnaround in nurse managers. More than ever, and whenever possible, **nurse managers should gather to mentor one another, share challenges and solutions, and have fun**. Collegiality among nurse managers has several benefits including:

- Moral support
- Mentoring and individual or group coaching
- Minimizing the opportunity for staff to play one practice setting or manager off against another

Trust in the Organization

While events associated with organizational change may challenge a nurse manager's ability to trust the workplace, each must choose to either move forward with his or her own measure of blind trust or go through the motions and join the ranks of the cynics and naysayers possessing just a dollop of paranoia. Consider the following actions for promoting trust in your workplace:

- Take time to reflect on your own actions that inspire and inhibit trust.
- Reflect on your experience of betrayal in the workplace. Name your feelings.
- Expect people to be trustworthy and most likely they will be.
- Conduct a conversation with staff about behaviors that build and betray trust. (See the discussion guide "Creating Respectful Workplace Relationships" in the Appendix.)
- Lead a discussion with staff about the importance of trust in practice, with patients, and among peers.
- Bring the topic of trust building forward for discussion at the middle management or senior leadership table.

TRUSTWORTHY BEHAVIORS OF SAVVY NURSE MANAGERS

The following inspiring and trust building behaviors by nurse managers will help create a place where staff members want to work.

- Recognize your own strengths and limitations and value the strengths of others.
- Trust others.
- Learn, grow, and change to become both a teacher and a learner.
- Lead by example; be there (staff cannot follow if you are not present).
- Take a leap of faith and lead into the unknown.
- Always tell the truth.
- Give others a chance to lead, make decisions, and make mistakes.
- Communicate, communicate, and, by the way, communicate!
- Own up to your mistakes.
- Be willing to laugh at yourself.
- Always speak positively about others and never discuss staff members in front of other staff.
- Model an attitude of harmony at work.

WORKPLACE CHARTERS

A workplace charter is an excellent tool to for reinforcing standards of positive relationships and elaborating how staff members will work together. Some workplaces have a code of conduct that achieves the same end, yet the language hints at being antithetical to caring and compassion. **A workplace charter is a document developed by staff that is influenced by their unit mission, vision, and values,** and identifies acceptable behaviors for anyone working in the practice setting. Introduced at orientation, charters become a tool for measuring the quality of staff's relationships.

Charters may include one- or two-line statements about any number of behaviors deemed important, including how decisions are made, treating all individuals with dignity and respect, maintaining confidentiality, expectations around meeting attendance, and conflict resolution. Creating opportunities for conversations that will expand values statements into a workplace charter builds trust, strengthens staff collegiality, and minimizes feelings of powerlessness. A good segue into building a charter could be:

> We, the staff of ______________, commit to one another to work together in the following ways:

Once completed, it should be signed by everyone, dated, and reviewed annually.

A BACK-TO-BASICS PLAN OF ACTION

Creating a plan of action built on the platform of your unit's mission, vision, and values, an environment of trust, and a workplace charter brings order to chaos during the organizational change process (or at any other time). Depending on its magnitude, change creates temporary or long-term disruption to staff. Recognizing this, a plan that addresses minimal expectations regarding the quality of care, workplace relationships, and accountabilities grounds staff in their work life reality, giving them a measure of peace. Adopting a three-pronged approach to shaping the plan, nurse managers ensure that the patient remains at the center, staff members maintain their standards of practice and code of ethics, and the practice setting is meeting its clinical mandate.

DEVELOPING A BACK-TO-BASICS PLAN FOR CREATING YOUR WORKPLACE FUTURE

Significant operational and clinical issues emerge during organizational change, and chaos, in stealth mode, can erupt before you know it. Creating an informal or business plan helps keep you and staff stay on the path of patient-centered care and professional practice, identifying and managing operational challenges and ensuring a collaborative, values-driven partnership. Using the headings of professional practice, workplace relationships, and organizational accountability, the following framework identifies hot spots and potential strategies that may prove helpful. Feel free to create your own categories and goals.

Professional Practice

1. **When task-focused care dominates professional nursing practice and the nursing process appears nonexistent, nurse managers must step in and assess care demands and care provision, identify gaps, and provide necessary resources.**
2. **The therapeutic relationship is considered a major task with no time to complete it.**

   Discuss with staff what else patients might need in their care besides the physical tasks. (This depends on scope and the nature of the practice environment; however, registered nurses [RNs] should not be exclusively task or paperwork focused. If they are, you must step in to determine what is preventing them from working to full scope and take remedial action).
3. **The art of nursing is but a distant, vague memory in the minds of many nurses.**

   Help staff reflect on what aspect of their care reflect the artful part of nursing and why.
4. **Care plans remain unwritten and in locked in a nurse's head.**

   Tell staff that this situation is nonnegotiable because the legislation says so. Show them a copy of the legislation that requires RNs to develop a plan of care. To top it off, show them their standards.
5. **Many nurses do not consider themselves knowledge workers.**

   At every opportunity, help staff link their practice to theory and evidence and standards. If they cannot do this, find out why. You might both have a problem.

Workplace Relationships

1. **You sense an undercurrent of tension in staff relationships.**

   Lurk! Be there around the desk, shuffle papers, listen and observe. If staff members wonder why respond with, "It is my job to be present and this helps me to understand better when I am here with you and not in my office." Be curious and ask questions, but listen more than you speak. Once you have an idea about what is happening, deal with it immediately.
2. **Articulating professional identity continues to challenge staff.**

   Have all staff do the exercise of developing their professional "15-second elevator speech." It is fun and inspires respect. Begin with, "My role as a registered nurse is to. . . ." (Do not list tasks.) Time it, memorize it, use it everywhere, especially with patients.

3. **Fear in the workplace.**

   This is a tough one, but it has a very powerful negative influence on quality of care and relationships. If you have a bully among staff, you must deal with them. If you choose not to you become a bystander and are not meeting your leadership standards. You have no choice.

4. **Self-compassion is virtually unknown among nurses.**

   Sometimes staff members blame themselves for things beyond their control. They try to be all things to all people and when they believe they have failed, they suffer guilt. Debrief specific situations with them, and talk about what they might do to help themselves. Most nurses would benefit from a conversation about self-compassion (an agenda item for a staff meeting?).

Organizational Accountability

1. **Working to full scope is difficult or impossible to achieve due to organizational barriers.**

   Identify what is not happening in care that is essential and why it is so. Talk to staff and formulate a plan to take forward to the next level of management. Specifically identify how these gaps in care are having an impact on expected patient care outcomes, emphasize the implications for staff, and offer suggestions for remedying the situation. Be creative in your approach. Write a formal memo to back up your statements. Report to staff and keep them updated. (Keep your regulatory body in mind as you reflect on practice implications.)

2. **Nurse managers receive little organizational support related to managing professional practice and leadership development.**

   Since most nurse managers do not have formal education to support their management practice, it behooves organizations, state boards of nursing, and provincial bodies to ensure the leadership is there to help staff do what is expected. Lobbying the organization to support nurse or clinical management professional development is a good investment in the future. Nurse managers can lead this awareness.

When staff members are engaged in this plan they begin to own their practice and their place in the organization, and see authentic nursing leadership in action.

FAST FACTS in a NUTSHELL

Summary

- Developing a practice setting mission, vision, and values statement aligns staff members with the "big picture," creating a sense of purpose, connecting them to a sense of participating in meaningful work and contributing to the greater good.
- Trust is foundational to relationship building.
- Charters are only relevant if they are regularly used to reinforce and guide professionalism in practice and healthy workplace relationships.
- Formulating a back-to-basics approach to care ensures a measure of stability in the practice setting by supporting staff in resolving issues that impact the quality of care and their work lives.

REFERENCE

Oakley, E., & Krug, D. (1994). *Enlightened leadership: Getting to the heart of change*. New York, NY: Simon & Schuster.

16

Got Staff Meeting Nightmares?

Managing Awesome Opportunities

Staff meetings are an amazing medium for facilitating change. When staff groups have meaningful and positive conversations with one another, they strengthen their professional and collaborative relationships. Yet, how many times have you heard staff members leave a meeting and comment, "Well that was a colossal waste of time!" How do you structure staff meetings that inspire staff to attend? This chapter will provide you with tips on how to create meetings that will engage staff and encourage them to assume ownership for their outcomes.

In this chapter, you will learn:

1. Information about how to create conversations that matter
2. Strategies to inspire staff from apathy to action
3. How to manage communication at staff meetings

TURNING AROUND THE *TITANIC*

Do you sometimes feel as if you are on a sinking ship when it comes to staff meetings? Is attendance plummeting? Is scheduling a staff meeting becoming more difficult, getting staff to attend harder, and holding staff attention taking on nightmare proportions?

In an era when time is a precious commodity, information overload is the new "normal," and demands on staff are never ending, scheduling a staff meeting is not an act of whimsy. **Staff meetings must pack a punch by being worthwhile, interactive, and productive.** If you are scheduling staff meetings and no one attends, it is time to make changes.

Luring staff nurses from the bedside or practice setting is difficult due in part to their work ethic and the belief that staff meetings interfere with patient/client care. In fact, "patient/client care" is the number one reason given by staff for not attending a meeting or leaving before it is over. While this is sometimes true, it serves as a ready excuse to avoid sitting through meetings characterized by "bobblehead" behavior and the belief that "nothing is happening" or "nothing ever changes."

"WHAT IF . . .": THE REAL VALUE OF STAFF MEETINGS

What if staff meetings became:

- An important opportunity in a safe place to talk to colleagues about things that matter?
- A medium for personal and professional transformation?
- A vehicle for strengthening workplace relationships?
- An opportunity for nurse managers to deepen their understanding of staff members, identify "hot spots," or create teachable moments?

When meetings are linked to professional development, opportunities to strengthen workplace relationships, and improve professional practice and quality of work life, staff members will come.

CONSIDERATIONS FOR SCHEDULING A STAFF MEETING

The need to schedule a meeting will vary with each practice setting. The most important considerations are:

- What is the purpose of the meeting?
- How will the meeting fit with the mission and vision of your practice setting?

- What do you want to accomplish?
- In building the agenda, what opportunities exist for interactive staff learning, conversations, problem solving, or relationship building?

PLANNING THE MEETING

- **Develop an agenda by seeking input from staff and adding items you want to bring forward.**
- **Define your purpose: Nice to know, need to know, need your ideas.**
  - **If the purpose is "nice to know," they won't attend.**
    If the meeting is "FYI only," you may want to consider another approach (e.g., a note in a communication book, e-mail, text message, or memos on the back of the bathroom door). Get creative about messaging.
  - **If the purpose is "need to know," they may attend.**
    If the purpose is to share information about an issue and receive feedback regarding the impact or their overall reactions, then schedule a meeting.
  - **If the purpose is "I need your input or feedback," they will attend.**
    When there is opportunity for new learning or a requirement to receive creative input from staff about how to manage a change, develop a new idea or process, or resolve an issue, staff are likely to attend.
- **Align the purpose of the meeting with your mission and vision.**
  - **Mission matters.** How does the meeting complement or enhance your mission? Is it an opportunity to learn about a new process to improve care or strengthen the quality of workplace relationships to enhance communication among team members? Tell the staff how the meeting furthers achievement of the mission and meets their needs for quality improvement.
  - **Value the vision.** How will the meeting help you and staff members move toward achieving the vision for your clinical practice setting?
- **Determine what you want to accomplish.**
  While planning the meeting, in your head, answer the question on the minds of your staff that will determine their attendance: "What's in it for me if I attend?" They may actually

get excited about attending a meeting that will be of benefit to them. The "What's in it for me?" question creates interest and peaks their curiosity.

- **Create opportunities to learn, converse, and relate.** Build in the opportunity for discussion among and between staff members during the meeting. For example, if there is a particular issue that requires staff input, do the following:
  - Divide the entire group into smaller groups.
  - Provide each group with questions to guide their discussion.
  - Have each group record notes highlighting their discussion.
  - After 15 to 20 minutes, have each group provide feedback to the larger group.
  - Make notes of key points on a flip chart.
  - Develop an action plan in which staff members volunteer to take responsibility for specific tasks.
  - Schedule a follow-up meeting or session.

IMPORTANT SUMMARY TIPS FOR GREAT STAFF MEETINGS

- Keep them short (no more than 1 hour).
- Always have a timed agenda with staff input.
- Make them timely (scheduling a meeting after the fact spells disaster for trust building). Preferably schedule them ½ hour before and after the shift change period.
- Always start and end on time.
- Reinforce staff's identified values to guide the meeting process, such as "respect."
- Stay on topic and curb sidebars.
- Create meaningful and timed small-group conversations and large-group feedback.
- Use a flip chart to capture key points identified by staff (this reinforces that you have heard them).
- Develop an action plan that staff takes responsibility for and identify a completion date.
- In wrapping up, state the key points of the meeting and the takeaway message(s).
- If you have a sense of humor, use it.

- If at all possible, and you have not already done so, try to develop your facilitation skills. They will serve you well in other situations.

FAST FACTS in a NUTSHELL

- Effective facilitation of a staff meeting ensures positive communication processes and outcomes.
- Staff meetings that are fun provide welcome relief from daily pressures, are more productive, and strengthen relationships.

MANAGING COMMUNICATION

- When staff engages in sidebars, interject with, "I notice that some of you are having fascinating sidebar conversations. It is important to hear everyone's ideas, so I am asking that you respectfully listen to you colleagues, okay?" If this does not work, try, "Yo! Listen up!"
- Continuously scan the group for negative nonverbal communication such as eye rolling, elbow jabbing, and facial expressions of sarcasm. (These behaviors require your follow-up ASAP).
- When the discussion gets off topic try the following: "It appears that we are off topic. We can continue the discussion later, after the meeting; add it to the next agenda; or I can follow up with you later." Then, get back to the topic at hand.
- Use your knowledge of therapeutic communication techniques to reinforce your staff's contribution to the conversations.
- If you are delivering "need-to-know information," capture the key points in a bulleted format to hand out to staff at the end of the meeting.
- Conduct a "check-out" before wrapping up by asking each staff member one of the following:
  - "What is your takeaway or key message from this meeting?"
  - "What did you learn from today's meeting?"
  - "Does anyone have any suggestions for how we can improve our next staff meeting?"

Summary

- Regular staff meetings keep staff informed and promote collaborative practice and relationship building.
- When nurse managers facilitate successful meetings, they have the opportunity to build leadership capacity, inspire trust building, and role-model excellence in communication.

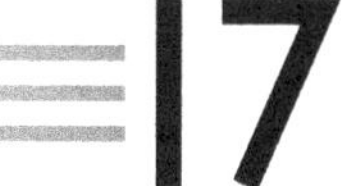

From Workplace to Community

Managing Connectedness

Whether your practice setting is a nursing unit in a busy hospital, clinic, department, outpost, or the community, you may have noticed that staff expresses a sense of isolation or disconnectedness frequently represented in the comment, "If only others knew what we really do here." How do you, as nurse manager, help staff make connections and build new relationships within the larger organization and setting in which the health care service is delivered? This chapter will help you to help your staff bridge these organizational gaps.

In this chapter, you will learn:

1. The value of promoting staff connectedness beyond the walls of the practice setting
2. How to encourage relationship-building capacity among staff members
3. Tips for managing staff opportunities for connectedness

DOWN WITH SILOS; UP WITH RELATIONSHIP BUILDING

In addition to managing the generation gaps, nurse managers must also help staff build relationships by managing relationship gaps

within the practice setting, the organization, and the community. Years ago, nurses tended not to focus on what was happening in the organization beyond the four walls of their practice setting. Nurses generally concerned themselves primarily with their own unit-based issues. Today, this type of thinking can be hazardous to a nurse's professional relationship health! Our relational economy requires organizations to strengthen the quality of workplace relationships to facilitate internal and external collaboration and organizational effectiveness.

THE BAD NEWS AND THE GOOD NEWS

The bad news is that many nurses now experience strong feelings of isolation and a sense of not feeling valued by others in the organization. These feelings may shed light on the powerlessness that so often accompanies the victims of organizational change or reflect oppressed group behavior.

The good news is that today, through a slow process of organizational osmosis, **nurses are learning more about the work of the organization**, how their practice setting complements that work, and the overall organizational impact on the well-being of the communities in which they serve.

Cross-pollination is occurring, as nurses participate with other staff members on organizational committees. In-patient nurses are teaching in the community. In a variety of practice settings, staff members are conducting "open houses" to showcase their work. Staff nurses are frequent members of organizational recruitment teams. The better news is that, for the most part, nurses love it! Participating on local committees becomes a launching point for participation at national and international forums, extending the nursing influence in health care planning and decision making.

A BLESSING AND A CURSE

Most everything has an upside and downside. As staff are inspired to spread their organizational wings into domains once considered the nurse manager's responsibility, staff nurses are conducting conversations and making decisions that occur outside their practice setting. This can be both a blessing and a curse. On one hand, nurses may enhance relationship building. However, taking nurses beyond their comfort zone with little experience or coaching in organizational (potentially political) relationships may require some nurse managers to engage in "damage control." Consider this as a natural part of the learning process; one in which you are willing to extend trust and consider mistakes as opportunities to learn. The purpose is to facilitate professional development. The benefits of facilitating relational growth opportunities for nurses include:

- Broadening staff members' individual and collective professional perspectives.
- Building leadership capacity when staff members represent their practice settings.
- Creating opportunities for expanding your staff's organizational learning regarding the culture, politics, and relationships that influence the health care setting.
- Facilitating two-way communication between frontline staff, the organization, and the community, and vice versa.
- Increasing staff autonomy through direct involvement in decision making.
- Positioning staff to positively influence professional practice organization-wide and beyond.

FAST FACTS in a NUTSHELL

- Facilitating connectedness creates opportunities for personal and professional growth through new learning, new conversations, and new experiences that promote excellence in service or care delivery, collaborative practice, and positive quality of work life.
- The process of connectedness and strengthening relationships begins when nurse managers move out of their comfort zone by becoming more visible across the organization and beyond. In doing so, they broaden their influence to effect change and model leadership. Furthermore, when they delegate staff to an organizational committee they are sending the unspoken message, "I trust you, you can do this," thereby strengthening their interpersonal connectedness!

INFLUENCING CONNECTEDNESS: CONDUCT A SELF-AWARENESS CHECK

- How connected are you to the larger organization? Do you lead, follow, or get out of the way? Are you a lemming or an organizational maverick?
- Do you participate in, speak up about, initiate, or lead the introduction of innovative ideas at the organizational level?
- What profile do you have in the community?
- Staff members are likely to follow your lead. If you are not connected then it will be difficult to inspire your staff. On the other hand, if you are too connected, spending most of your time away from the practice setting, staff members may resent your absence and resist your efforts to involve them.

MANAGING THE BALANCE CHALLENGE OF CONNECTEDNESS

Learning to broaden your connections while maintaining stability in your practice setting is a delicate balancing act. Consider it as an art form and a work in process. Learning where, when, and how best to make connections beyond your workplace occurs through trial and error. It depends on the level of professional autonomy among your staff members, and on your own comfort level at being able to "leave them on their own." Sounds a bit like parenthood!

Trial and Error

In attempting to broaden your connections and model connectedness, it is easy to become overinvolved in external committee work, projects, and planning exercises. Be prepared to step back if staff members begin to complain that you are "never there." In their heads staff are saying, "There's no way I'm spending my time away from my patients working on committees. I'll never have time be with my patients. That's not what I signed up for."

Level of Professional Autonomy Among Staff

When staff possesses a high level of professional autonomy, you may be able to spend more time away from your workplace to advance your connectedness, spread your professional influence, and demonstrate formal leadership at a higher level.

When staff members have less professional autonomy and require more supervision, coaching, and role-modeling, they have a higher need for your visible presence. This may require you to pick and choose your connection opportunities according to your availability. For example, your practice setting may be less hectic in the afternoon, freeing you up for committee participation.

Your Comfort Level

Severing the proverbial umbilical cord by breaking away from your practice setting and forging new relationships in advancing professional connectedness may feel uncomfortable at first, and you may to want to retreat to your familiar turf.

- Resist the urge to turn tail and run! It will get better.
- Give yourself permission to feel your way along as you journey down this new road. This is not unlike the feeling you may have had as a new parent leaving your child with the babysitter for the first time.
- Help staff members to understand your absence by reporting to them about what you are doing, what you are learning, and how your involvement benefits their practice.

TIPS FOR MANAGING STAFF OPPORTUNITIES FOR PROMOTING RELATIONSHIP BUILDING CONNECTEDNESS

There are countless opportunities for connecting beyond your workplace that include:

- Modeling connecting behaviors, such as becoming an in-house speaker on specific topics, inviting staff in the organization to come and see the work of your practice setting, writing an article, leading an initiative, or asking members of the community to participate on a practice setting committee

- Supporting opportunities for staff to lead initiatives that may have an impact on the organization, such as time off for participation on committees
- Facilitating conversations about the value of staff connecting beyond the practice setting
- Educating staff about your committee involvement by taking them with you to a meeting (this depends of course on the nature of the committee meeting, prior approval, and support from the committee as a whole)
- Encouraging and supporting staff to conduct an "open house"
- Encouraging and providing time for staff to write about their practice for publication in a professional journal or an organizational newsletter
- Encouraging staff members to invite staff from other departments to your workplace to talk about how they can support one another or strengthen their working relationships
- Meeting with individual nurses to talk about their aspirations for influencing practice beyond the level of their practice setting. (Some at first may have no desire whatsoever. Keep an eye on this attitude as a developmental opportunity for your future attention.)
- Creating structures for staff to provide feedback on their off-unit professional activities
- Providing opportunities for leadership development within the practice setting, such as team leading, chairing the occasional staff meeting, clinical teaching, attending nursing practice development meetings, or taking a staff nurse with you to meet with another department representative
- Advocating for staff nurse representation on committees that would not normally even consider their presence
- Inviting staff to participate in presentations to senior leadership
- Looking for opportunities in the community for staff nurses to "strut their stuff" as, for example, providing health teaching in schools, facilitating focus groups, running for political office, participating in career days, and attending and presenting at conferences on local, national, and international levels
- Coaching or facilitating the acquisition of resources to support nurses' ability to speak up and speak out

Summary

- Connectedness is foundational to building trust, respect, collaborative interprofessional relationships, quality care, and organizational success. Nurse managers can model and lead the way in extending this competency beyond the bedside and practice setting into the broader community and beyond.

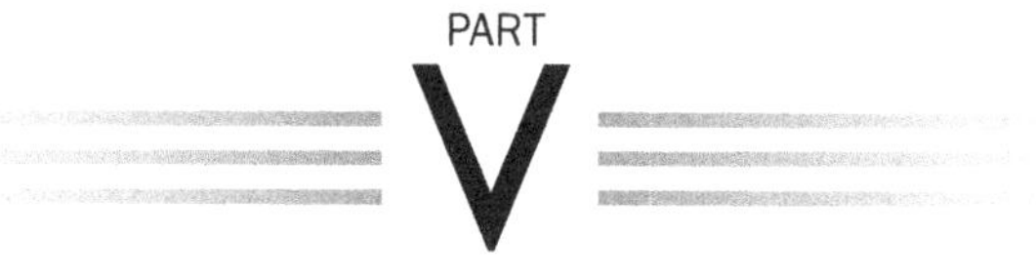

A Call to Action—From Surviving to Thriving to Recovering the Art of Nursing

Tips and Tools for Managing a Changing Workplace

18

Recovering the Lost Art of Nursing

A cunning group of masterminds known as the "the evil-doers," a notorious bunch consisting of the "thieves of time," "organizational skulduggeries," and the villainous "them" (aka the "fiscal restrainers") are turning the nursing profession upside down! They are systematically stealing one of nursing's most precious gifts to the world of health care—the art of professional caring. Absence of the art renders nurses technicians of care, efficiently moving from one task to another. Left in the wake of staff with little to no time for building therapeutic relationships, patient care becomes an item on a to-do list that receives a check mark at the end of shift.

Nurse managers, this chapter is your urgent call to action to muster your personal and professional leadership resources, on behalf of patients, and join together with staff to remove system barriers and recover the art of nursing. Warning: Apparently, "evil-doers" are specifically targeting therapeutic relationships, compassion, absence of "presence," professionalism, and identity confusion. Time is of the essence!

In this chapter you will learn:

1. The need for urgency behind the call to action
2. The clues of a covert art theft presence
3. Strategies for reclaiming the art of professional practice

IDENTITY THEFT

Despite all the decades of circuitous discourse, mountains of scholarly articles, nursing theories, and educational preparation, the term *art of nursing* leaves many nurses struggling to describe its meaning within the context of their professional identity. Nursing practice is a symbiotic relationship between the art and science of professional care. One cannot exist in isolation from the other. Nurses are inclined to connect the art of nursing with terms such as *compassion, caring attitudes, the therapeutic relationship, presence, professionalism, advocacy,* and *competence,* otherwise known as the "soft or caring side of nursing." The science seems more linked to the procedural, technical skills and competencies associated with the physical tasks of care. In today's frequently chaotic and frenzied practice settings, nurses face challenges that force many of them to choose between these tasks or the relational aspects of care. Feeling overwhelmed and backed into a corner by time constraints and the physical demands of care, they make a judgment call, defaulting to Maslow's hierarchy in attending to physical safety needs first, and fueling patients' and families' perceptions that "the nurses here are too busy to spend time with me" (also expressed as, "I don't want to bother the nurses"). At the end of shift, staff members feel exhausted, guilty, disheartened, and inadequate. The "evil-doers" have scored another hit!

RED FLAG MOMENTS

The greatest threat to the disappearance of the art of nursing lies with the perceived "big three": (1) time, (2) fiscal restraint, and (3) failure of the system to support a full staff of nurses, so those employed are working at full capacity.

ASK NOT WHAT NURSES ARE SAYING, ASK WHAT THEY ARE NOT SAYING

When you hear staff say, "We don't have enough time" or "We don't have enough staff" (despite being at full complement), and your desk is piled high with "inadequate staff" notices, be mindful of your response. While the tendency is to fix this problem with a knee-jerk response, step back for a moment and ask what is not being said. The comments and requests may be a call for help to deal with a significant practice issue larger than nurses believe they have the power to influence or control. Underlying this behavior is a deeper emotion left unexpressed: *Fear.* Their practice is threatened and they need a champion—and you're it! Consider the following utterances, and what each implies:

- "The system is failing me. I can't do what is required."
- "I'm not meeting my standards."
- "Why can't my manager do something?"
- "I'm frustrated and angry and feel bad about my practice."
- "The patients are suffering because my hands are tied."
- "I could do so much more but time won't allow it."
- "Why did I become a nurse? All those years of education and expense and I can't practice what I learned to do."
- "The theories we learned can't influence care delivery in a system like this."
- "How long will it take for the system to figure out they are paying nurses a lot of money to do a lot less than their scope requires?"
- "I'm outta here!"

This is a red flag moment and cause for deep concern. When the art of professional nursing practice is MIA (missing in action), it is your job to draw attention to the fact and lead the recovery initiative. Action is not an option because you are accountable (according to the standards) for the overall quality of care and care delivery model. You have the evidence of research to support interventions to support nurses working to full scope.

A second red flag presents itself during budget season when senior leadership becomes preoccupied with the bottom line, requiring you to analyze care requirements, staffing mix, and hours of care. It is fair to say that at this time management is caught between a clinical rock and a hard place, with everyone scrambling to fight for every dollar and defend why their department, practice setting, or staff deserves to be saved from the chopping block. With the focus inclined toward viewing the costs of nursing staff as opposed to their value added in quality care outcomes, fiscal decision making defaults to cutbacks of nurses (expensive) rather than equating nursing excellence to organizational success. Few senior leaders have witnessed firsthand what nurses working to full scope actually do. Communities are now beginning to "see the light," recognizing the health benefits to individuals and communities as a whole in having nurses work in independent and collaborative practice. Acute and long-term facilities appear to be slower off the mark.

FAST FACTS in a NUTSHELL

- Without the art of nursing, nursing practice becomes a mechanistic series of tasks. The evidence of a scientific, humanistic, and compassionate approach to professional care can quickly evaporate, increasing the possibility of negative care outcomes and, in some cases, replacement of nurses with less-expensive personnel.

The third red flag is one the nursing profession would prefer to remain unfurled. This flag signals a problem with how nurses choose to practice and the nurse manager's expectations of practice. Nursing culture is well entrenched in the tendency to blame someone or something for nurses' difficulties. The moment we attempt to identify the part we might play in creating the issue, cries of, "You're blaming the victim!" are heard far and wide. This victim behavior has to end. We must first look to ourselves to fix what is within our control and influence. In short, if the art of nursing is disappearing, it is our job to retrieve it. Our standards of practice require it, our professional licenses hinge on it, and our patients depend on it (although they may not be quite clear about what to expect from professional nursing care unless we tell them). Here's a deep thought: Would trial lawyers accept a system that prevented them from going to court? Would engineers tolerate not having time to survey a piece of land before building a road, and would surgeons consider it okay to operate on a patient without completing an assessment or developing a plan? The answers to these questions point the way forward for nurses to take uncompromising action.

FAST FACTS in a NUTSHELL

- We must do everything in our power to preserve and maintain the art of nursing as integral to professional nursing practice.
- To allow it to slip away alters the profession at its deepest level, potentially posing a threat to the viability of the nursing role in health service delivery.

Controlling the attitudes and behavior of others is not within our power. Influencing may be. We have power to take some responsibility for our current situation and control our future actions. We can also create an opportunity for change and create a new reality. Identifying the art of nursing as a rallying point can inspire staff nurses and nurse managers to work together in proclaiming that professional nursing practice is not exclusively about task-focused care, and that we will no longer accept the disappearance of the art of nursing. Nursing is a complex blend of expertise in caring for the physical, bio-psychosocial, and spiritual needs of others throughout the life cycle. These essential elements of professional practice are mandated by the law.

RECOVERY STRATEGY

It is important to recognize that different practice settings have varying needs. Some areas, such as emergency departments and intensive care units, are high task areas while others, such as mental health settings, may focus less on tasks but require high relational aspects of care. One size does not fit all. Yet the requirements for nursing assessments, developing a plan of care, coordinating care with other health care providers, implementing interventions, and evaluating care outcomes are a requirement of all.

The following framework offers a potential model for points to ponder and actions to consider in recovering the art of nursing. Each practice setting has its own culture, staff members at varying stages in their careers, and a nurse manager with his or her own experiential status. Feel free to tweak the plan to fit your specific needs. The principal goal is for you to reestablish the art of professional practice in order to meet comprehensive nursing care requirements, standards of practice, and nurses' professional satisfaction. Consider these steps:

1. Be Present

- Be there (in the practice setting) in body and spirit!
- Determine the degree of urgency related to the need to recover the art. When nurses are exhausted, focusing their energies exclusively on the physical tasks, and referring to patients as numbers or diagnoses, the urgency level is considered high.
- Inform staff of your role in supporting their practice and that you are there to get a true handle on their situation.
- Invite conversations and questions.
- Keep your office door open.

2. Connect the Professional Dots

- Invite staff to a meeting and share your observations. Convey the message that their current reality (be specific in describing it) must change (reinforce reality) for a number of reasons, including meeting their standards, patient care outcomes, and job satisfaction. Convey support, not blame; empathy for and recognition of their struggles; confidence in the necessity for change; and determination that this will happen.
- Remind staff that yesterday is history; we cannot change what went before, but we can create a better professional future.
- Help staff understand how their current circumstances are connected to external realities that have a direct impact on their practice and on areas they have the power to influence and control.
- Enlist their support to work together to create a win–win future for all: their patients, their practice, and the organization.
- Enlist support from your nurse leader.
- Keep your office door open.

3. Create a Compelling Vision

- Together, reflect on your clinical mandate, needs of your patient population and the specific role nurses will play in meeting their health care needs.

- Discuss and develop a clear professional practice vision.
- Use every opportunity to facilitate conversations that connect nursing actions of staff and *their* vision. Create opportunities to communicate your unit's vision verbally and in writing to your senior nurse leader and beyond.
- Keep your office door open.

4. Do Your Research

- Assign staff or ask for volunteers to research the current literature related to the identified hot spots.
- Invite research and conversations of models of nursing care and evidence-based practice that support the specific nursing care required for your practice setting.
- Evaluate the clinical effectiveness of available organizational tools to support clinical practice.
- If necessary, review the tools nurses use to initiate the nursing process to determine whether or not they are effective. If they are not, then be prepared to defend the need for revising or replacing the existing tools to support improved professional practice.
- Leave your door open!

5. Develop a Plan

- Establish a pilot project for a specific length of time.
- Enlist the help of a clinical educator or create, with staff, a pre-project and post-project attitudinal survey of staff about their professional practice environment.
- Invite informal leaders to lead specific areas.
- Identify priorities based on observed hot spots and sources of dissatisfaction with current care processes related to demonstrating the art and science of professional practice, and the meeting of standards.
- Communicate your plan to relevant stakeholders and invite feedback.
- Focus on the fact that this is a staff-driven initiative, a requirement of their professional nursing practice, and fulfillment of an important aspect of your nurse manager accountability and responsibility.
- Establish timelines. Create a visual grid.

- Schedule regular progress updates, communicate outcomes, and elicit feedback.
- Keep your door open!

6. Stay Focused on the Goal

- Slow and steady wins the race. Keep your eye on the goal to influence and create the conditions for nurses to practice their art within their scope of practice. Expect resistance and challenges never before experienced for you and staff members. Try to take them in your stride. As your care delivery changes to meet professional practice standards, educating others and communicating why changes are occurring is critical. Remember, this is not a harebrained scheme to create more work. It is essential for a retrieving a professional world in decline.
- Expect and talk about your wins and losses along the way, mistakes and opportunities to learn, self-doubts and vulnerabilities, and the importance of maintaining focus. You are the wind at the staff's professional backs.
- Meditation helps.
- Keep your door open.

7. Continuously Evaluate

- Make changes as necessary and build on the knowledge of what works well and what does not. Link current research to validating observations and developing a "go forward" plan (e.g., "Several studies have reported improved [patient outcomes, quality of care] with ________. Let's try this. . .").
- Develop simple evaluation tools for staff and patients.
- Share your evaluation outcomes with others, what steps you are now taking, your new goals, and the renewal, revitalization, and professional satisfaction and sense of control over practice staff are beginning to experience.
- Revise your goals as you achieve your clinical milestone plan.
- Review and revise written protocols to reflect changes in nursing practice and processes.
- Is your door still open?

8. Build on Your Successes

- Look for opportunities to influence and inspire replication of this process in other practice settings.
- Discuss lessons learned and how organizational success may be enhanced by staff's efforts.
- Seek opportunities for you and staff to tell their professional story, to reinforce the necessity for organizational change if they are going down the task-focussed road, and to give evidence of improvements in quality of care, staff morale, and job satisfaction.
- Since the absence of the art of nursing most frequently reveals itself in patient and family complaints, talk about patient, family, and staff positive feedback (it will become evident).
- Close your door, catch your breath, open your door to success!

FAST FACTS in a NUTSHELL

Summary

- Vanquishing the "evil-doers" and leading the recovery of the lost or disappearing art of nursing may be your greatest challenge to date.
- It will require the best of what you have to offer: your prowess at organizational leadership, your sound knowledge of professional practice, and your ability to facilitate relationship building, organizational change, and operational success.
- Your call to action is clear. The time for change is here. If you do not act, who will? Now more than ever the patients, the nurses, and the profession urgently require your leadership.

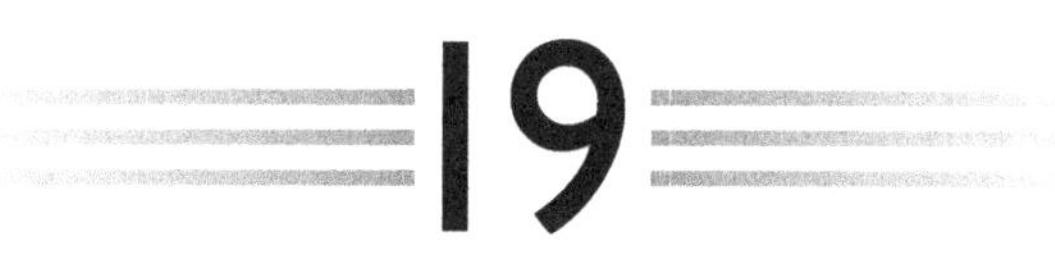

Top 10 Fast Facts for Thriving in a Changing Workplace (and 12 More for Managing It!)

Thriving in a changing workplace does not happen by chance. In a thriving workplace, nurse managers possess high levels of self-awareness, set the tone for excellence in practice, and require values-driven healthy workplace relationships to achieve a healing environment and therapeutic practice setting. When nurse managers thrive, so do staff. The Top 10 Fast Facts included in this chapter offer key strategies for thriving as opposed to just surviving on both a personal and a managerial level.

In this chapter, you will learn:

1. Top ten *personal* tips for thriving in a changing workplace
2. Top twelve *management* tips for creating a thriving workplace

TOP 10 PERSONAL TIPS FOR THRIVING IN A CHANGING WORKPLACE

1. Choose Your Attitude, Wisely

You have the power to choose your attitude. When you choose a positive attitude, you change the quality of your future.

2. Take Care of Yourself.

If you do not take care of yourself, who will? You cannot adequately lead and manage a thriving workplace and create a happy home life if you do not have harmony at work. Get help if you need it. You are, after all, only human! Start small by taking relaxing baths, slowly build up to Mediterranean cruises!

3. Get Your Priorities Straight

At the end of the day, what really matters most? Reflect on your values and determine if your personal values match your workplace values.

4. Pick Your Battles; You Can't Win Them All

Ask yourself this: "Is this the hill I want to die on?" Try to identify what you can control or influence. If you cannot do either, move on.

5. Remember the Three R's: Respect for Self, Respect for Others and Respect for Your Organization

Reflect on the actions required to demonstrate R-E-S-P-E-C-T. Do you require being treated with respect? How respectful are you of others?

6. Focus on Today. Yesterday Is History; Tomorrow Is a Mystery

Today is all that you have.

7. "Be the Change You Wish to See" (Gandhi) and Inspire It in Others

Walk the talk; do what you say you will; treat others the way you wish to be treated. Live your values!

8. The Best Way to Predict Your Future Is to Create It

Determine what you want in your future, and then set about to create it!

9. Cultivate or Resurrect Your Sense of Humor

Well-placed humor is both infectious and therapeutic. If you have a sense of humor, use it. If you do not, that's okay too. Appropriate laughter in the workplace becomes conspicuous by its absence. When staff members say, "We never laugh here anymore," it is time to find ways to lighten up. Grab a teaspoon and prepare to administer a dose of levity. After all, laughter is good medicine!

10. Don't Wait for Others to Change; You Go First!

If you are holding your breath waiting for others to change their behavior, two things will happen:

1. They will not change, and
2. You will turn blue!

TOP 12 MANAGEMENT TIPS FOR THRIVING IN A CHANGING WORKPLACE

1. Begin With a Journey of Self-Discovery

Being self-aware is a great teacher. Plan time for self-reflection. Forgive yourself and others. Learn about power, influence, and getting political. Consider exploring the concepts of mindfulness, presence, and self-compassion. Staff members will reap the benefits as well.

2. Authentic Leaders Have Nothing to Hide

They inspire trust. Always tell the truth; staff members know when you are not being upfront and will "fill in the blanks" with what *they think* is missing. Before you know it, the grist for the organizational rumor mill is churned out at warp speed.

3. Expect Respect for All

Require respectful behavior from and toward all staff members, physicians, patients, families, and visitors.

4. In Crises, Look for Opportunities; In Opportunities, Expect Snags

Most change creates reactions ranging from the good to the okay to the ugly. Snags may be blessings in disguise. Look for the possibilities.

5. Create a Place Where Staff Wants to Work

Creating a practice environment grounded in excellence begins with you. Set the tone by clearly stating expectations framed around patient care outcomes, hire the right staff, inspire staff through regular communication and feedback, and challenge staff to soar both personally and professionally.

6. Create Opportunities for Fascinating Group Conversations and Inspired Dialogue

Staff meetings are one of the most powerful tools in the nurse manager's toolkit. Craft agendas that excite and energize, invite conversations and laughter, and they will come. If you supply refreshments, staff will beat down the door!

7. Breathe Life into the Standards of Practice

When staff performance deviates from the standards of practice and staff members are not held accountable, they start on a slippery professional slope that can negatively affect the quality of care and work life. You cannot monitor adherence to the standards if you are not present in the practice setting to draw attention to them! If you are present you can assess staff's competence, identify their learning needs, and determine where they fit on the professional practice autonomy scale.

8. Periodically, Step Back and Monitor the Quality of Staff Relationships, Levels of Wellness, and Staff Risk for Burnout and/or Compassion Fatigue

Ever increasing clinical, technical, and relational demands are placing greater numbers of staff at risk for burnout and compassion fatigue. Familiarize yourself with the symptoms and consider providing an informational session to staff as a means of promoting self-awareness and professional wellness. Keep in mind your own level of vulnerability in the face of these insidious conditions.

9. Build Your Workplace Mission, Vision, and Values to Guide Professional Practice and Quality of Work Life

Staff members do well when they are confident that there is a good organizational fit between their skills and the work that is required. They also need to know how their workplace fits into the context of the organization, as well as the guidelines and actions that govern behaviors to accomplish what needs to be done. A practice setting mission, vision, and values statement is a compass that gives direction to the workplace and all who work there.

10. Develop a Workplace Back-to-Basics Plan, Your Pathway to the Future

This plan become the template for how you and your staff will move forward together to achieve your mutual goals. Furthermore, the plan will reinforce a mindset of thriving no matter what is happening, helps staff focus on what really matters in terms of patient care, and helps them with professional accountability and professionalism in practice.

11. Deal With Behavioral Problems

Although this is one of the most uncomfortable tasks that nurse managers must face, dealing with untoward behavior is never optional. The longer the behavior goes unchecked, the greater the potential for destroying workplace relationships, quality of work life, and quality of care.

12. Facilitate the Development of the "15-Second Elevator Speech" for All Staff Positions

This is step one in collaborative and professional practice approach.

FAST FACTS in a NUTSHELL

Thriving in a changing workplace requires you to give yourself three gifts:

- The gift of time to reflect
- The gift of a positive attitude
- The gift of courage to create your future

Appendix: Conversation Guides and Activities

Tools to Inspire

This section will offer you a variety of discussion guides and activities to use to inspire conversations, ignite creativity, and promote engagement of staff to take ownership for their professional practice, managing change, and creating a healthy workplace.

In this section, you will learn:

1. To inspire creative conversations that will promote staff ownership of work life issues
2. To capture staff's ideas on paper that can be foundational to staff-generated action plans
3. To create relational learning opportunities among staff through meaningful conversations when they gather together to discuss mutual concerns, generate ideas, learn from one another, and develop creative strategies over which they may have influence and/or control

Feel free to adapt these tools to fit your unique situation. When staff follows the guides and writes down comments from their conversation, the written word takes on greater significance for them. This recorded conversation then serves as a point of reference to create action plans and benchmarks for evaluation of staff initiatives.

POSTCARD FROM HOME

Purpose

This exercise helps staff identify what they believe to be the ideal qualities of a place where people would want to work. From this you can extract a mission, vision, and values for your practice setting.

1. Divide staff into groups of three.
2. Ask them to pretend that they have a friend working in another country and they want the friend to consider returning home to work in your practice setting. Ask staff to complete the following:

> Dear___________
>
> I am writing to you to entice you to return home in order to work in our practice setting____________. I believe that this is the most professionally fulfilling workplace that I have ever worked in because:
>
> Please give it some thought.

Have each group read its cards to the whole group. Look for common threads between the groups and their content. Ask for volunteers to collect the postcards and prepare a draft for the remaining staff to critique. Revise again until staff agrees with the revisions.

CREATING OUR VALUES

Purpose

To help staff develop values that they feel ownership of and that will govern their workplace relationships.

Equipment

- Flip chart at front of room (1 flip chart page per group)
- 1 piece of paper per person

Instructions

1. Ask staff to form small groups of three or four.
2. As you stand next to a flip chart ask staff to call out one-word values that they believe to be important in the workplace. Write them down in list format on the flip chart (no more than 15).
3. Ask each person to pick five that he or she feels are most important, write them down on a piece of paper, and then discuss the choices in his or her small group. Have one person in each group record all the choices in a list on one page. When a value is repeated, make a check mark next to it.
4. Each small group then selects its top three values. Record these on your flip chart to create a list. Look for duplicates.
5. Create a new consolidated list and ask each staff person to come forward and check off his or her three top values. Select the three or four values that received the most check marks.

BACK TO OUR FUTURE, PART I: EXERCISE

Purpose

This powerful and creative exercise allows groups of staff to intermingle and collaborate in a fun way. It is designed to get them "on the same page," to bring "baggage" to the surface in a nonthreatening way, as well as to share ideas.

Equipment

- Flip chart at front of room (1 flip chart page per table group)
- 1 package of crayons

SAMPLE FLIP CHART PAGE

1. Where were we (in the good ol' days)?	2. Where we are now.
3. Where do we want to be?	4. How we're going to get there.

Instructions

1. Instruct the groups to divide the flip chart page into four sections with each quadrant labeled as shown.
2. Ask the groups to draw with their crayons their responses to the headings.
3. Rules for artwork: No people or stick figures are allowed. Words are to be kept to a minimum. Animals, birds, insects, flowers, objects, anything else nonhuman are allowed. Have fun! No spying between groups!

Process

1. Allow 20 to 30 minutes for groups to complete the artwork.
2. Observe the group dynamics and the laughter!
3. Invite people to the front of the room to explain their pictures.
4. After everyone has presented, ask the following questions:
   a. In your table group: What did you hear? What did you see? What did you learn?
   b. In the large group: What did you hear in your group? What did you see? What did you learn?

The lessons this exercise teaches include:

- In Quadrant 1: Initially, staff glorifies the "good ol' days"; then realize, maybe they were not so good.
- In Quadrant 2: Staff sees that today's workplace relationships are a mixture of strengths and needs for improvement. They recognize that most people want to make things work.
- In Quadrant 3: The pictures usually depict a workplace utopia where staff is happy and relaxed. Themes of vacationers on a Caribbean island, ants, and geese flying in unison are often depicted.
- In Quadrant 4: Pictures commonly include hands together, hearts, collaboration, technology, and money.

Key Messages From This Exercise

Following the large-group discussion, summarize the following key messages:

1. Respect for diversity: Despite their differences they achieved their goal.
2. No one has all the answers: Together they are better.
3. Results oriented: They demonstrated their ability to complete the task in a relatively short period of time.
4. Laughter: Because the sound of laughter was so prevalent, the task was much easier to complete. They still have the ability to laugh, and having fun at work is not only okay, it is doable!
5. Creativity: They discover that working together generates creativity.
6. Collaboration: They listen respectfully to one another.
7. Task completion. They came together, made decisions in a short period of time, and got the job done well.
8. Diversity: Despite differences in age, culture, and experience, they focused on the same goal and achieved the desired results.
9. Judgment was suspended.

BACK TO OUR FUTURE, PART 2: FOLLOW-UP CONVERSATION

Once staff members have completed the artwork exercise, instruct them to think about Quadrants 3 and 4 and complete this discussion guide.

Instructions

In order for us to adapt to our changing workplaces and create our futures, each of us will have to learn, grow, and change.

Some things that we may have to learn include:

1.

2.

3.

Things that will help us to grow personally and professionally include:

1.

2.

3.

Strategies that we can use as individuals to help each other to manage change could include:

1.

2.

3.

Our nurse manager can help us manage change by:

One suggestion for the union to help members manage change would be to:

CREATING RESPECTFUL WORKPLACE RELATIONSHIPS

One issue that we have in our workplace relationships is living the value of *respect*.*

1. It is important to address this issue because:

2. We all have a role to play in creating healthy, respectful workplace relationships. We believe that:

   a. Individuals could demonstrate respect by doing the following:

   b. Managers could demonstrate respect by doing the following:

   c. Staff could demonstrate respect by doing the following:

   d. As a whole, the organization could demonstrate that all relationships are founded on the value of respect by:

   e. Union and management could together demonstrate respectful relationships when they:

*Substitute any value, such as accountability, compassion, excellence, collaboration, and so on.

Bibliography

Barker, J. (1988). *Discover the future: The business of paradigms*. St. Paul, MN: ILI Press.

Beer, M., & Eisenstat, R. (2000). The silent killers of strategy implementation and learning. *Sloan Management Review, 41*(4), 29–40.

Bennis, W. (1999). *Managing people is like herding cats*. Provo, UT: Executive Excellence Publishing.

Bridges, W. (1991). *Managing transitions: Making the most of change*. Reading, MA: Perseus Books.

Fisher, H. (1999). *The first sex: The natural talents of women and how they are changing the world*. New York, NY: Random House.

Freire, P. (1997). *Pedagogy of the oppressed*. New York, NY: Continuum.

Fry, B. (2007, May 3). Workplaces must do more than treat bullying symptoms. *Halifax Chronicle Herald*.

Fry, B. (2011). *A nurse's guide to intergenerational diversity*. Canadian Federation of Nurses Unions. Ontario, Canada: Plantagenet.

Fry, B. (2013a). Get the job done: Straight talk about scope of practice. *Canadian Nurse, 109*(3), 32–33.

Fry, B. (2013b). Power up your leadership: Straight talk for nurse managers. *Canadian Nurse, 109*(5), 32–33.

Fry, B. (2013c). Straight talk: Why we must do better. *Canadian Nurse, 109*(1), 32–33.

Fry, B. (2014). Straight talk: Creating our future. *Canadian Nurse, 110*(4), 12.

Government of Canada. (n.d.). *Work/life balance and new workplace challenges: Frequently asked questions*. Retrieved June 15, 2006, from http:www.canadian-network.ca

Hankin, H. (2005). *The new workforce: Five sweeping trends that will shape your company's future*. New York, NY: AMACOM.

Hutchinson, M., Jackson, D., Vickers, M., & Wilkes, L. (2006). Workplace bullying in nursing: Towards a more critical organizational perspective [abstract]. *Nursing Inquiry, 13*(2), 118–126.

Marshall, E. (1995). *Transforming the way we work*. New York, NY: AMACOM.

Maurer, R. (1996). *Beyond the wall of resistance*. Austin, TX: Bard.

Nazarko, L. (2000). Bullying and harassment. *Nursing Management, 8*(1), 14–15.

Oakley, E., & Krug, D. (1994). *Enlightened leadership: Getting to the heart of change*. New York, NY: Simon & Schuster.

Peplau, H. (1988). *Interpersonal relations in nursing*. London, UK: MacMillan Education.

Reina, D., & Reina, M. (2006). *Trust and betrayal in the workplace: Building effective relationships in your organization* (pp. 128–140). San Francisco, CA: Berret-Kohler.

Roberts, S. J. (1983). Oppressed group behavior: Implications for nursing. *Advances in Nursing Science, 5*(3), 21–30.

Roberts, S. (2000). Development of a positive identity: Liberating oneself from the oppressor within. *Advances in Nursing Science, 22*(4), 71–82.

Russell, S., & Shirk, B. (1993). Women's anger and eating. In S. P. Thomas (Ed.), *Women and anger* (pp. 170–185). New York, NY: Springer.

Short, R. (1998). *Learning in relationship: Foundations for personal and professional success*. Bellevue, WA: Learning Technologies.

Stuart, G., & Laraia, M., (2000). *Principles and practice of psychiatric nursing* (7th ed.). St. Louis, MO: Mosby.

Sullivan, E. (2004). *Becoming influential: A guide for nurses*. Upper Saddle River, NJ: Pearson–Prentice Hall.

Thomas, S. (2003). Anger, the mismanaged emotion. *Medsurg Nursing 12*(2), 103–110.

Thomas, S. (2004). *Transforming nurses' stress and anger: Steps toward healing anger* (pp. 15–32). New York, NY: Springer.

Thomas, S., & Jefferson, C. (1996). *Use your anger: A woman's guide to empowerment*. New York, NY: Pocket Books.

Thomas, S., Smucker, C., & Droppleman, P. (1998). It hurts most around the heart: A phenomenological exploration of women's anger. *Journal of Advanced Nursing, 28*(2), 311–322.

Vaill, P. (1996). *Learning as a way of being: Strategies for survival in a world of permanent white water*. San Francisco, CA: Jossey-Bass.

Index

Printed in the United States
By Bookmasters